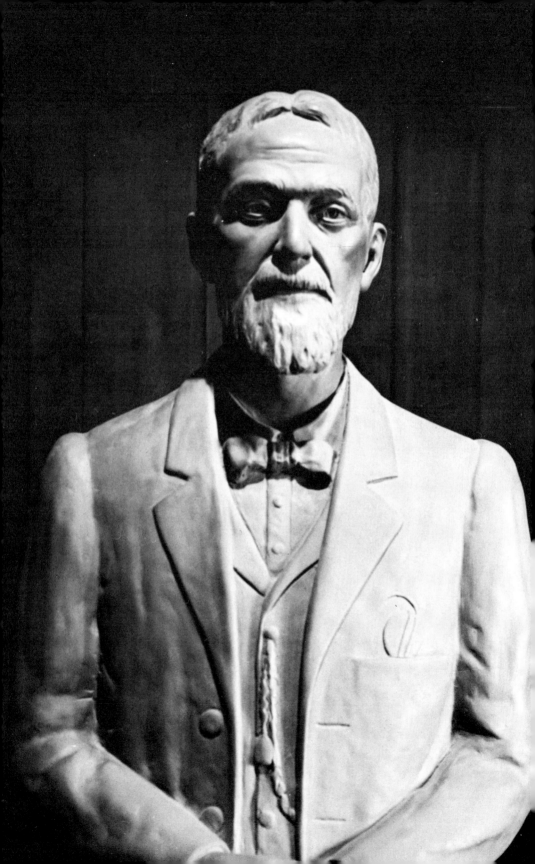

OSTEOPATHIC MEDICINE: AN AMERICAN REFORMATION

GEORGE W. NORTHUP, D.O., F.A.A.O.
AMERICAN OSTEOPATHIC ASSOCIATION
CHICAGO, ILLINOIS 60611

To my father,

Thomas L. Northup, D.O.,

more than a doctor:

a physician

PREFACE

Since the first college of osteopathy had its beginning in Kirksville, Missouri, in November 1892, the osteopathic profession has had the responsibility of describing itself to physicians and patients alike. Born on American soil in the nineteenth century, the osteopathic profession has grown with the twentieth century in both size and importance. It is an accepted member of the health professions of this country.

Medicine as a subject is not easy to discuss. Its language is not a universal one and, because of this, misunderstanding develops. This applies to osteopathic medicine as well. Being a relatively new development in the long history of medicine, osteopathic medicine has not always been well understood by either medical professionals or the public.

The purpose of this book is to present a summary of osteopathic medicine. Philosophies defy definition, and osteopathic medicine is essentially a medical philosophy. Its first exponent, Andrew Taylor Still, described it as a philosophy for medicine and one which he conceived "to give the medical world a start in a philosophy that may be a guide in the future." It is the development of this philosophy that constitutes the major objective of osteopathic medicine today.

Andrew Taylor Still was an American and as such conceived of osteopathic medicine as an American reformation. Emerging at a time when medical practice did not have the advantages since produced by modern science, he found much to be desired. Faced with the failures of the then "modern medicine," Dr. Still borrowed from some neglected philosophies of the past and made new applications to the practice of medicine in his day. His story and the story of osteopathic medicine constitute an important and evolving process in contemporary medical life.

This book does not purport to be a scientific thesis. It is merely one man's attempt to provide all those who have sufficient interest to open these pages to obtain a bird's eye view of osteopathic medicine, its history, and its theory. It is not an "official" interpretation approved by a roll-call vote of all osteopathic physicians. It is unashamedly an interpretation and admittedly an epitomization. However, we believe that it is a reasonably clear picture of the past and present of this profession. It is respectfully submitted to all whom it may concern.

George W. Northup, D.O., Editor
American Osteopathic Association

FOREWORD

A medical reformation, even though historically oriented, by its very nature requires an interpretation of a movement rather than a chronicle of it. Although much has been written about the beginning and the development of osteopathy as a reform movement in medicine, the matter is not broadly understood. In the frontier states of Kansas and Missouri a hundred years ago, communication and medical education were conducted on a much less formal basis than today. Manners of expression were metaphorical and rustic, and life was vigorous. Few have had the ability to interpret to the modern-day reader the thinking and methods of operation of Dr. Still and his contemporaries, products and producers of late nineteenth and early twentieth century Americana.

Dr. Northup has been able to draw a picture with words that not only clearly portrays the reform movement but also explains the need from which it sprang and follows its course through varying climates. The text was developed in 10 articles published separately in HEALTH magazine, but each "part" blended with the next so smoothly that no continuity was forfeited in the multiplicity of issues in which the installments appeared. Because of the volume of requests for reprints, it was deemed advisable to compile the material in a single publication.

I believe that *Osteopathic Medicine: An American Reformation* provides us with an important addition to osteopathic literature.

True B. Eveleth, D.O.
Executive Director
American Osteopathic Association

CONTENTS

I

HISTORICAL
ROOTS OF
OSTEOPATHIC
PHILOSOPHY

Centuries of medical history have fashioned a tapestry on which are woven the chronicles of current concepts and practices of medicine. To say that the philosophy of osteopathic medicine *began* with the pronouncement of Andrew Taylor Still, its founder, ignores the historical roots of the osteopathic profession. They can, indeed, be traced to the teachings of the great Greek physician-philosopher Hippocrates, who stressed that man must be treated as a whole.

Man has always been concerned with his health, his welfare, and his survival and has recognized disease as a threat to all three. For the important task of safeguarding his health, since prehistoric time man has assigned particular people the duty of managing and treating the discomforts of mind and body.

High in the Pyrenees Mountains of Spain is the famous Trois Freres Cave. On its walls is probably the oldest known portrait of a "medicine man." Those who have observed this work of art say that it closely resembles the African "witch doctor" known to our twentieth century generation. Authorities in anthropology agree with historians of medicine that the earliest "doctors" considered health and disease to be connected with either magical or religious powers. Superstition and ritualistic practices followed naturally.

WITHIN OR WITHOUT?

Primitive man thought of disease as arising from either of two sources. The one cause of disease was thought to be some outside morbid influence that entered the victim. It was intimately related to hexes, forces of nature, and the evil desires of outside human energies.

1

A contrasting viewpoint developed purporting that disease was some abstraction of the soul within the body of the victim. Therefore, two diverse "theories" of health and disease evolved, and, from these basic premises in medical history, many theories and concepts were developed, either supporting or contradicting the "inside" and "outside" theories of medicine.

Supporters of these apparently contrasting philosophies varied from witch doctor to witch doctor, from one ethnic group to another, and from one civilization to the next. It was not until the era of Greek predominance in medical history that an attempt was made to organize into schools of philosophical thought a practical application. So-called modern medicine has its birth with the development of the Hippocratic school of medicine.

Hippocrates is said to have been born on the island of Cos, close to the coast of Asia Minor, in 460 B.C. He became a physician and teacher of great skill and is called the "Father of Medicine." From his students he extracted a pledge concerned chiefly with medical ethics and including promises not to cause injury willfully or to divulge confidence. Known now as the Hippocratic oath, it is still taken by many physicians before they enter practice.

RESPECT FOR NATURE

Before his death in approximately 377 B.C., Hippocrates lived a long and fruitful life and succeeded in establishing a base for the medical teaching of his time. He founded the teachings of his school of medicine on the belief that, although the causes of disease could orginate outside *or* inside man, "it is our

"The Temples and Cult of Asclepius" (©1957, Parke, Davis & Company)—*The Grecian Temples of Asclepius were the nightly destinations of sick pilgrims from 500 B.C. to 500 A.D., hoping that the god of medicine would heal them or prescribe remedies. Stone or terra cotta images of afflicted parts that healed were hung on the temple walls by grateful patients.*

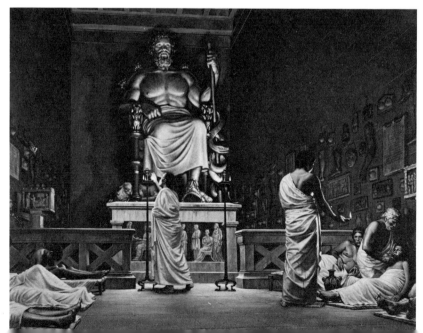

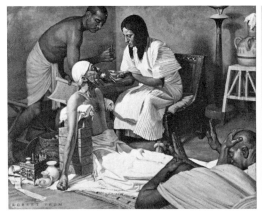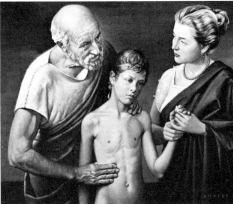

Left: "Medicine in Ancient Egypt" (©1957, Parke, Davis & Company)—An Egyptian physician of the Eighteenth Dynasty (1500-1400 B.C.) ministers to a patient, who is supported by a "brick chair." The patient shows signs of lockjaw, and the physician's assistant holds a scroll containing directions for treatment. Right: "Hippocrates: Medicine Becomes Science" (©1958, Parke, Davis & Company)—Hippocrates, the "Father of Medicine," is shown as a kindly physician examining a young patient and comforting a worried mother sometime late in the fifth century B.C.

natures that are the physicians of our diseases." In a collection of Hippocratic writings called "Aphorisms," he reminded his students not to meddle with nor hinder nature's attempt toward recovery.

In *A History of Medicine,* Douglas Guthrie sums up the Hippocratic philosophy well: "The work of Hippocrates is not a mere matter of historic interest. The idea of focusing full attention on the patient, rather than on scientific theories of disease or elaborate laboratory tests, was revised by Sydenham, Boerhaave, and today it is again engaging the attention of some of the best minds in medicine. We cannot be too frequently or too forcefully reminded of the fact that our natures *are* the physicians of our diseases. The physician and the specialist, whatever his field, should study the entire patient and his environment, and should view disease with the eye of the naturalist. This is the message of Hippocrates, as fresh today as it was 2400 years ago."

DISSENTERS AT CNIDUS

Regardless of the dominance of Hippocrates' approach in Greek medicine, it was too philosophical for many of his medical colleagues. Some had joined together to work out a more "practical" approach to medicine and develop a school to promote the approach of a specific cause for *each* disease. This antinomy of philosophy traced itself to the inner conflicts of prehistoric "medicine men." Was disease an *outside* malevolent intruder, or was it a morbid condition that existed within man himself?

While the Hippocratic school emphasized the study of the health of man as

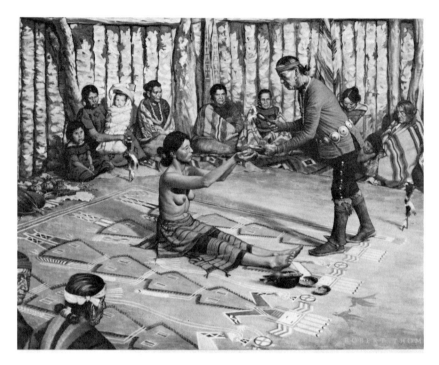

"Primitive Medicine" (©1957, Parke, Davis & Company)—Sand-painting ceremonies of American Navaho Indians are beautiful examples of primitive medicine. Family and friends gather in a medicine "hogan" and join in the nine-day ceremonies in which sand painting plays a major role. The "singer" (medicine man) sings, prays, manipulates magico-religious artifacts, and administers herb preparations to the patient, spectators, and himself.

an individual, integrated unit, the rival school at Cnidus, a nearby peninsula, steered its attention away from man toward the disease, the afflicter of man. This theoretical battle, with its prehistoric origins, wedged a major conflict into medicine that persists still.

It is interesting to study the history of medicine and to watch the ebb and flow of these apparent conflicts of medical thought. Basically, osteopathic medicine and its physiological principles are supporters of the Hippocratic approach. Although it borrows from both the Hippocratic and the Cnidian, the emphasis is clearly on Man rather than the individual diseases that afflict man.

PHYSICIANS IN HISTORY

Hippocrates has been emulated down through the ages, and certain other physicians in history who have specially adhered to his teachings or developed his point of view have been linked with his name. For example, early in the Christian era there lived a famous Chinese physician, Chang Chung-King, who is referred to by historians as the Chinese Hippocrates. He inaugurated a study of disease based on patient observation rather than separate theories for each disease, a radical departure from the annals of Chinese medical history. Sixteen hundred years later, Thomas Sydenham (1624-89) made similar observations and was dubbed the English Hippocrates by medical historians.

Dr. Sydenham entered practice at a time when medicine was a hodgepodge of rival, conflicting systems. Known for his astute clinical observations, this great English physician took the doctor of his time away from textbooks and existing fanciful theories back to the bedside of the patient. His admonition, "Young man, go to the bedside; there alone can you learn disease," typifies his attempt to reform the medical practices of his day to a Hippocratic philosophy. The genius of Thomas Sydenham was not recognized during his lifetime, but later received just acclaim.

As we approach, in time, the twentieth century, medical historians often describe Samuel Hahnemann (1755-1843), a German doctor and the founder of homeopathy, as a physician who developed the Cnidian principle of disease to an extreme. Dr. Hahnemann developed a system of medical treatment that is often associated with the use of drugs in extremely small dosages. However, the key principle of homeopathy seemed to lie not so much in the absurdly small dose as it did in the selection of the drug.

Despite his critics, there is little question that Dr. Hahnemann added greatly to the knowledge of the action of pharmaceutical agents. Despite his apparent dedication to the basic Cnidian philosophy, he inadvertently supported the Hippocratic approach. By effectively starting a countermovement to the over-dosage of medicinal agents that have long since been discarded, in his lifetime

"Sydenham and Clinical Medicine" (©1959, Parke, Davis & Company)—*Thomas Sydenham (1624-1689) is called the English Hippocrates because of his brilliant straightforward clinical observations. Here, his simple attire contrasts with the flamboyant costume of his friend John Locke, physician-philosopher, who often accompanied him on rounds.*

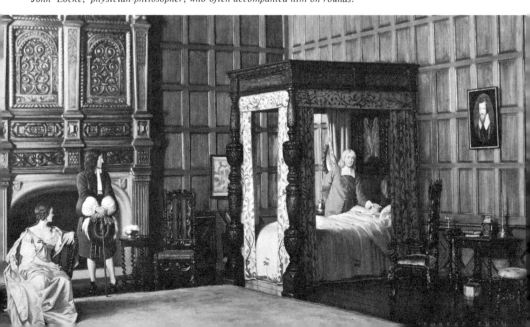

he removed stress from the over-drugged bodies of patients that was beneficial both to health and to medical understanding. Despite the apparent extremist viewpoint of Dr. Hahnemann and his followers, he made his contribution to medicine.

Slightly before the time of Hahnemann, one of the greatest teachers of eighteenth century medicine and perhaps of all time was developing in Europe. Hermann Boerhaave (1668-1738), the son of a Dutch country pastor, was described as being "poor in money but pure in spirit." As a junior lecturer in medicine, the young physician attracted many students, and with his acceptance of the chair of botany in medicine at Leiden in 1709, his fame became worldwide. People from all over Europe and America attended his lectures. Without question, Dr. Boerhaave was the most popular teacher and fashionable physician of his day. He, like many predecessors, chose the Hippocratic philosophy of medicine as his guide. He placed the patient in the center of the stage and encouraged patient observation rather than theoretical argument. Dr. Boerhaave's respect for Sydenham was so great that it is reported that he always raised his hat when the name Sydenham was mentioned.

OSTEOPATHIC MEDICINE FOLLOWS NATURALLY

To those of orthodox medical heritage it is difficult to accept Andrew Taylor Still (1828-1917), the founder of osteopathic medicine, as a man in the Hip-

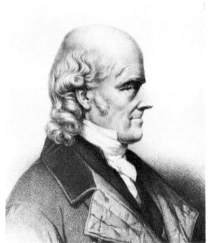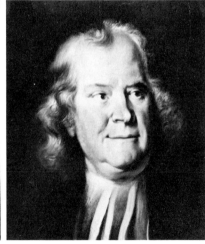

Left: Samuel Hahnemann (1755-1843), the German physician who founded homeopathy, is described by medical historians as a physician who developed the Cnidian principle of disease to an extreme. (Bettmann Archive). Right: Hermann Boerhaave (1668-1738), celebrated physician and teacher of the eighteenth century, was guided by the Hippocratic philosophy of medicine in encouraging patient observation over theoretical argument. (Bettmann Archive).

pocrates, Sydenham, and Boerhaave tradition. To be sure, Still was a rough-hewn frontier doctor in the midwestern United States, developed in the crucible of turbulent times and steeled by the flame of personal tragedy. Like his more sophisticated and "acceptable" predecessors, however, Dr. Still was a man dissatisfied with the *status quo* of medicine. He believed that the drugs of his day were either inert therapeutic agents or toxic burdens imposed upon an already diseased body. Like Hippocrates, Sydenham, and Boerhaave, Still turned to a study of man to lead him toward the secrets of health and mysteries of disease. He was one of the first in his time to note that if one studied the attributes of health he might be better able to understand the processes of disease.

Dr. Still was an eccentric nonconformist. He was an individualist who pursued his beliefs with intensity. He believed that Man should be studied as a total unit. He believed that within the body of man were those substances necessary for the maintenance of health and, hence, if properly stimulated, might also be the substances necessary for the cure of disease. He did not believe that disease was strictly an outside agent inflicting its evil on the body but considered instead that it was a normal body response to an abnormal body situation.

In his search for the positive quality of health, he came to a startling conclusion. He discovered, as others throughout the history of medicine had noted, that the skeleton and its supporting muscles and ligaments were subject to certain mechanical laws and therefore were the objects of stresses and strains. Within his philosophy was the concept that man, among his other attributes, was a mechanism subject to mechanistic law.

Dr. Still observed, through careful study of the patient, that when joints, restricted in motion due to mechanical locking or other related causes, were normalized, certain disease conditions improved. He also noted that not only was there a local response to pain in the body structure but he believed that he noticed an improvement in the function of other systems of the body as well. If there were a unity to the body and an interrelationship to its many parts, why exclude the musculoskeletal system, with its muscles, bones, ligaments, tendons? Could it be that this portion of the body, representing its greatest mass of tissue, had been relatively ignored through the thousands of years of medical history? Could it be that the proper function of these parts of the body and their effect on the nervous system and the circulatory system might be important factors in health and disease?

Dr. Still believed that they were. However, like many of his predecessors, particularly those who followed a Hippocratic philosophy, his views were far from universally accepted. The physician voiced his belief to outstanding professors of medicine in the Midwest, and he was rejected as being a crank. However, convinced of the soundness of his theories, Dr. Still, with the support of his friends, developed a school of medicine to teach and explore the Hippocratic philosophy and the significance of the musculoskeletal system in the health of mankind.

During Dr. Still's lifetime and to the present day, the basic physiological principles of osteopathic medicine and the term "osteopathy" have been focal points of medical controversy and debate. Overtones of medical politics have crowded the basic scientific issue. Yet, the soundness of the Hippocratic approach expressed in a different manner and leading to different observations through the work of these medical leaders continues like a golden thread through the history of medical science. Although the basic philosophy of osteopathic medicine, which provides the emphasis for the study of a relatively little understood and undertreated portion of the body, has been repeatedly demonstrated by the osteopathic profession, it has often been cast aside by the misnomer of "cult."

Truth can be camouflaged but it cannot be destroyed. Members of the osteopathic profession today are leaders in establishing the validity of the great medical tradition of the philosophy of the Hippocratic school. Recognizing the great need for the proper treatment of medical emergencies and disease episodes, osteopathic medicine contends that there is more to health than the specific treatment of a "specific" disease. It is upon this foundation that osteopathic medicine stands and makes its contribution as a reform movement, in the Hippocratic tradition, to all of medical practice.

II

ANDREW
TAYLOR STILL

On August 6, 1828, in a log cabin three miles west of Jonesville, Lee County, Va., a son was born to Abram and Martha Still. He was named Andrew Taylor.

Not unlike Lincoln, Andrew Taylor Still was of humble origin. His father, a physician, minister, and frontiersman, ministered to the bodies and souls of his backwoods neighbors. The sturdy English-German background of his father and the Scottish heritage of his mother were to serve him well in the rugged frontier days ahead.

From Andrew's boyhood, the Still family was on the move. In 1834, when he was six years old, the Stills moved to New Market, in eastern Tennessee, where he and his two brothers attended an elementary school known as "Holston College."

In 1837, the elder Still was sent as Methodist missionary to northern Missouri. The trip there from Tennessee was made in seven weeks, with "two wagons, seven horses, and eight in the family." The family settled in Macon County, Mo., and for three years Andrew attended a typical frontier school. When he was 12 years old, the family again moved, this time to Schuyler County, Mo., but returned to Macon in 1845.

Conditioned by his environment, young Andrew became a close friend of nature, and spent many hours observing its wonders. In minute detail, and with an almost passionate fervor, he investigated the works of God's creation and, under his father's tutelage, became interested in the structure and function of things in the world about him. He found it to be a beautiful and awe-inspiring world, but its discords did not escape him. Disease and death were such frequent companions of the early settlers that it is little wonder that Andrew Taylor Still was drawn to things medical.

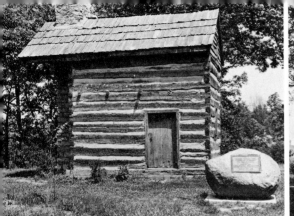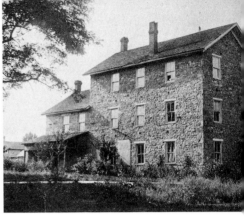

Left: The log cabin in which Dr. Andrew Taylor Still was born on August 6, 1828, was moved from Jonesville, Lee County, Va., to the campus of the Kirksville College of Osteopathy and Surgery and is preserved as an historical exhibit. Right: An early building of Baker University, founded in Baldwin, Kans., in 1858, was on land donated by Dr. Still and two of his brothers. It was here he wished to announce his medical concepts in 1874, but the University was closed to him.

As the son of a Methodist circuit rider who was also a country physician, the young man was appalled not only by the toll of disease but equally by the lack of knowledge concerning its cause and treatment. Such diseases as cholera, smallpox, and meningitis, rarely encountered today, were the scourges of the frontier. Entire families were ravaged by plague. It is little wonder that the sensitive mind of Still was stimulated by frustration. He developed the desire to serve his fellowmen with more efficient care than they were receiving.

IN THICK OF CONTROVERSY

To say that Still was destined to be a man of conviction is to understate. From his very young manhood, his political views were to keep him in the center of controversy. Life in Missouri placed him in a precarious position. Missouri was a "border state" with proslavery leanings, and along with his father young Still was an ardent abolitionist. A person of lesser character would have avoided controversy.

The elder Still was caught up in continuing conflict and the divided sentiments of his own church. In 1844, he was appointed as a missionary to the Shawnee Indians and with his family moved to Kansas. Two years later Andrew, then 18 years of age, married Mary M. Vaughn.

Andrew joined his father in the fight against slavery. In 1857, he was chosen by the people of Douglas County to represent them in the Kansas legislature. There, he quickly aroused the anger of the proslavery group. A segment of the Methodist Church known as the "New Church" made the claim that slavery was of divine origin. Its members believed that the Bible justified it.

Andrew's wife died in 1859, and late in 1860 he married Mary E. Turner.

The gathering clouds of America's Civil War broke, and young Still, a fervid supporter of Lincoln, enlisted in the Ninth Kansas Infantry, at Fort Leavenworth, in September 1861. In May 1862 he was commissioned captain of the 18th Kansas Militia, and saw active duty in this and other units. By the end of the war, he had risen to the rank of major. He was discharged in October 1864.

Still was to find out, however, that despite the North's triumph in battle, the people's problems were far from settled. As he later wrote:

"I was not long in discovering that we had habits, customs, and traditions no better than slavery in its worst days, and far more tyrannical."

It is interesting to note that years later, when Still founded the American School of Osteopathy, he declared the institution open to Negroes. He was one of the first of America's educators to provide such opportunity, but he found his liberal viewpoint unacceptable to many. He added to the controversy, which seemed always to surround him, by pleading for woman suffrage as well.

HIS MEDICAL EDUCATION

Following the end of the war, Still resumed his study of nature and of health and disease. His medical education was typical of his time. Much of it was by preceptorship, with some formal training. It is reported that before the Civil War he attended the College of Physicians and Surgeons of Kansas City, but that before he completed his course he left to enlist in the army. His training was similar to and probably better than that of many physicians of his time. With a father who combined missionary work with the care of the sick, Andrew had literally grown up in medicine. Even as he used the "remedies" of the period, however, his mind kept record of something that went back to his childhood. Apparently he had suffered from headaches. He wrote in his *Autobiography:*

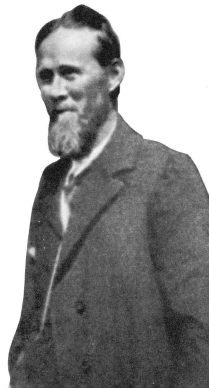

Dr. Still, a familiar figure in Kirksville, Mo., was known to all its citizens as he took his daily walks. He established the first college of osteopathy there in 1892, and died there in 1917 at the age of 89.

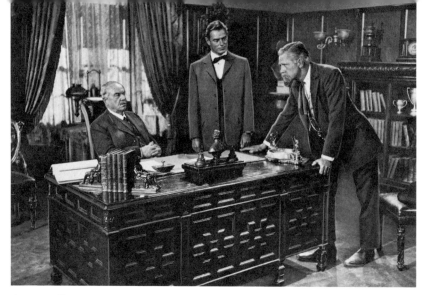

A scene in "American Doctor," a motion picture filmed under the auspices of the American Osteopathic Association, dramatically depicts Dr. Still's being refused permission to present his ideas at Baker University.

One day, when about ten years old, I suffered from a headache. I made a swing of my father's plow-line between two trees; but my head hurt too much to make swinging comfortable, so I let the rope down to about eight or ten inches of the ground, threw the end of a blanket on it and I laid down on the ground and used the rope for a swinging pillow. Thus I lay stretched on my back with my neck across the rope. Soon I became easy and went to sleep and got up in a little while with the headache gone. As I knew nothing of anatomy at this time [he was ten years old], I took no thought of how a rope could stop a headache and the sick stomach which accompanied it. After the discovery I roped my neck whenever I felt those spells coming on. I followed that treatment for 20 years before the wedge of reason reached my brain and I could see that I had suspended the action of the great occipital nerves, and given harmony to the flow of the arterial blood to and through the veins, and ease was the effect . . .

STUDY OF MAN

This experience pricked at Still's inquiring mind when, shortly after the end of the war, he began his practice of medicine. He was finding the medical theory and practice he was using to treat the sick totally inadequate, and totally unacceptable. The dissatisfaction he had felt during the war years mounted. Still was not a complacent man. He was held by the statement of Alexander Pope, "The proper study of mankind is man." Could it be that his homemade headache remedy might be a lead in developing a new and dynamic philosophy for all of medicine?

Textbooks offered no answers to Still's provocative questions. He turned, therefore, to the study of the body itself, the function of its organs, and the function of its structure. To provide himself with material for dissection, he exhumed bodies from the graves of Indians. As he later recorded, "A thousand experiments were made with bones, until I became quite familiar with the bony structure."

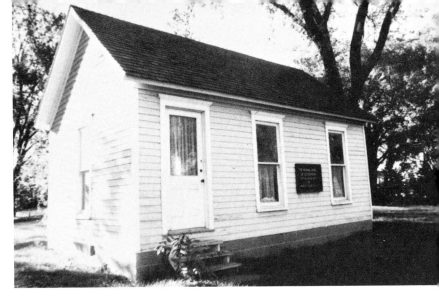

The frame structure that housed the first classes in osteopathic medicine is preserved on the campus of the Kirksville College of Osteopathy and Surgery. (Pat Patterson).

This sketch is of the frame cottage where the first college of osteopathy was founded in 1892. There were 20 students in the first class. The school is now the Kirksville College of Osteopathy and Surgery, one of the country's five training centers for osteopathic physicians and surgeons.

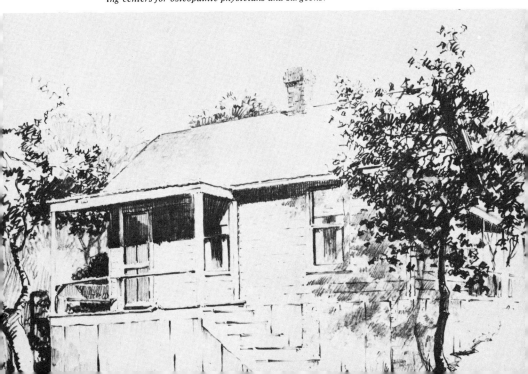

It was personal tragedy, however, that convinced Dr. Still that a higher order of medicine must be conceived. In the spring of 1864 a terrifying epidemic of meningitis, an inflammation of the covering of the brain usually due to infection, struck the Missouri frontier. Thousands died. Among them were three Still children, two of them his own and one an adopted child. Armed only with the medical knowledge of his day, Still sat helplessly by as death took his loved ones.

This personal tragedy served to drive him relentlessly on in his study of man. Slowly he began to develop the philosophy that was to occupy his mind for the remainder of his life. By 1874 he considered his concepts ready for presentation to the medical world. He felt that the time had come for their introduction into medical practice.

HELPED FOUND A UNIVERSITY

He chose Baker University in Baldwin, Kans., as the place for his presentation. In 1858 Dr. Still, his father, and his brothers had been a part of the founding of this university. They had donated the 480-acre tract of land that was to become the university campus, and much of the lumber for the early buildings was sawed in the 40 horsepower sawmill Andrew and his brothers helped erect for the purpose.

Yet when Dr. Still asked permission to present his ideas at the university, he was turned down. In spite of his generosity and that of his family, of his reputation as a good medical doctor, of his service in the Civil War, and of his record as a state legislator, the doors of the university he had helped found were closed to him.

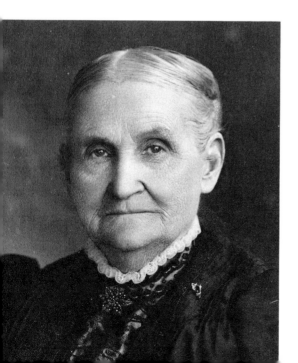

This photograph of Mary Turner Still, Dr. Still's wife, was taken in the late years of their life together.

This was a blow, but it was not a defeat. Dr. Still returned to Missouri, firm in his determination to continue to develop his ideas and to incorporate them into his medical practice. Later, his philosophy of medicine will be discussed more fully. It is now enough to say that through these years of study and contemplation he had come to the belief that man should be treated as a *unit*, that he cannot get sick in one area of his body without having other areas affected. He believed that:

Within man's body there is a capacity for health. If this capacity is recognized and normalized, disease can be both prevented and treated;

The structure of the body is reciprocally related to its function;

Progress can be achieved in the study of disease if first a study is made of health;

The body's musculoskeletal system—bones, ligaments, muscles, fascia, etc.—forms a structure which, when disordered, may effect changes in the function of other parts of the body. This effect may be created through irritation and abnormal response of the nerve and blood supply to other organs of the body;

The body of man is subject to mechanical disorder.

MANIPULATIVE THERAPY

Through experiment and clinical observation, Dr. Still developed the fine art of manipulative therapy, applied directly to the musculoskeletal system. He eliminated the use of many toxic drugs from his practice—in itself a health benefit to his patients.

Let us follow Dr. Still's own words: "I spent much time in the study of anatomy, physiology, chemistry, and mineralogy. During the winter of 1878 and 1879, I was called by telegram to my old home in Kansas to treat a member of a family whom I had doctored for ten years previous to my moving to Missouri. I treated partially by drugs, as in other days, but also gave osteopathic treatments. The patient got well."

More patients were treated in this manner, as success followed success. First, Dr. Still's fame grew. People from all over the United States flocked to the little town of Kirksville, where Dr. Still had settled. Second, and equally significant, as his fame spread he was attacked by his former medical colleagues as a "crank," "faker," and a man who had lost his reason. The persecution and abuse he received would have discouraged the most determined, but not Dr. Still.

Despite this opposition from the majority school of medicine, Dr. Still attracted the objective interest of many physicians. Eager to impart the results of his studies to qualified people, the Doctor soon found himself overwhelmed, first with his practice, then with the teaching of those who sought him out. His reponsibilities became greater than one person could bear.

FOUNDED A PROFESSION

His theories, rejected by the "modern medicine" of his time, had to be developed further. At no time did Dr. Still believe that his word was the final one. At no time did he attempt to establish restrictive scientific dogma. Admittedly eccentric and nonconforming, Dr. Still was humble concerning his discoveries. With the help of his sons and of doctors of medicine who had been attracted both by curiosity and the desire to learn, he founded the profession that is now known as osteopathic medicine.

The first formal classes for the teaching of osteopathic medicine met in Kirksville in November 1892, under a charter taken out in May of that year. A second charter was issued October 30, 1894, to the American School of Osteopathy. As stated in the corporation papers filed at Jefferson City, capital of Missouri, the objective of the school was "to establish a college of osteopathy, the design of which is to improve our present system of surgery, obstetrics and treatment of diseases generally, and place the same on a more rational and scientific basis, and to impart information to the medical profession, and to grant and confer such honors and degrees as are usually granted and conferred by reputable medical colleges; to issue diplomas in testimony of the same to all students graduating from said school under the seal of the corporation, with the signature of each member of the faculty and of the president of the college."

These "articles of association or agreement" testify that the osteopathic school of medicine from the first was considered to be a school of medicine

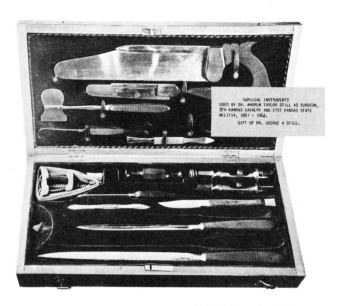

Dr. Still enlisted in the Union army in 1861, joining the Ninth Kansas Infantry at Fort Leavenworth. He was commissioned a captain aud rose to the rank of major, seeing service as a surgeon. The surgical instruments used by Dr. Still during the Civil War are on display, labeled as shown here, at the Smithsonian Institution in Washington, D.C. (Smithsonian Institution)

embracing all of the arts and sciences of medical practice. It was never a "non-medical school of medicine." It was a philosophy for all of medicine, gauged "to improve its practice."

MEDICAL WORLD OF THE TIME

In order to evaluate the magnitude of the mind of Dr. Still, it is appropriate to remember that the medical world of 1874 was only beginning to emerge from confusion. As told by Leon E. Page, D.O., in his book *The Principles of Osteopathy:* "The tubercle bacillus would not be identified for eight years. Lister, then in his prime, was trying to introduce antiseptic surgery against much conserative opposition. The use of diphtheria antitoxin and the x-ray would not be introduced for another twenty years. Pasteur, then fifty-four years of age, had established the germ theory of disease only ten years before. Osler, a young man of twenty-five was beginning his work as a professor at McGill University. Another twenty-five years would pass before Harvey Cushing would bring the first blood pressure instrument to the United States. Yet with none of these advantages, Still worked out a system of practical structural therapeutics which subsequent discoveries have progressively confirmed and never invalidated."

Andrew Taylor Still died in Kirksville on November 12, 1917. More than

5,000 osteopathic physicians were then in practice in the United States and abroad. There are now more than 13,000.

Today, Dr. Still would be called a liberal, both in politics and in medicine. It is little wonder that his theories and his personality evoked controversy. He was a complex man, and many of his writings are difficult to understand. They were written in the idiom of his day and contained many allegories. Unfortunately, latter-day historians have used the allegories as fact and have missed their purpose. In these times, the liberal views of Dr. Still are still opposed, politically and scientifically. Yet in a slow but inexorable progression, modern medicine confirms, without apparent recognition, the concepts of Andrew Taylor Still. Dr. Still did not present his philosophy as dogma, nor did he bind a profession rigidly to his views. As he states clearly in the Introduction to his book, *The Philosophy of Osteopathy,* his great desire was "to give the world a *start* in a philosophy that may be a guide in the future." It is this philosophy that is emerging in the development of osteopathic medicine today.

THE PROFESSION TODAY

Since Dr. Still, there have been many giants in osteopathic medicine. They have contributed much to its refinement and development. Today the osteopathic profession — with its hospitals, its educational institutions, and the far-flung activities of the American Osteopathic Association, headquartered in Chicago— serves the public health through the initial inspiration of this intrepid doctor and soldier who emerged from America's frontier.

III

THE UNITY
OF MAN

Andrew Taylor Still was not first in proclaiming the concept of the unity of man. He was, however, a pioneer in relating this fundamental principle to the *treatment* of disease. In advancing the precept of the whole man and its application in clinical medicine as one of its basic premises, osteopathic medicine set in motion an American reformation in the medical world.

Even prior to the advent of Hippocrates to the medical scene, thoughtful philosophers and physicians continually reminded their students that man must be considered in the completeness of his composite body. His physical body, his mind, and his soul were parts of a triumvirate that formed a unified human biological unit. This ultimately became one of the fundamental precepts in the school of medicine founded by Hippocrates.

This medical philosophy was opposed by the so-called "practical theorists," who contended that such a panoramic approach was too broad for practical application. Disease was considered to be something almost apart from the human organism. Too many physicians still view disease solely in its limited aspects as a malevolent impostor intruding upon and destroying the health of man.

At the time Still began to theorize, there were no philosophical principles to unite medicine. The approaches to the maintenance of health and beliefs concerning destruction through disease were diverse, fragmented, and empirical.

Down through the ages medicine has been considered a "science" that needed no philosophy. By Still's day, medicine had become a series of haphazard remedies, which in many cases were more destructive than the disease they purported to treat. Both the genius and the courage of Still rested on the fact that he stood practically alone in recognizing the futility of the then modern medical approaches and the prevailing need for the science of medicine to have a basic philosophy soundly founded on anatomical and physiological principles.

MANIPULATIVE THERAPY

In the course of his investigation, hampered by ineffectual medication and poorly developed surgical techniques of his day, Still developed manipulative therapy as a means of providing total body treatment. As important as the therapy was, it was but a means of expressing Still's basic philosophy for the treatment of total man. If, as Still believed, all of the various systems of the body were interrelated and interdependent, surely the musculoskeletal system could not be divorced from a consideration of the unity of the body. Fortunately, and sometimes unfortunately, manipulative therapy has been the hallmark of osteopathic medicine. It has been *fortunate* in the fact that manipulative therapy is a powerful and valuable method of treatment in the maintenance of body unity in health and in the prevention and treatment of its diseases. It has been *unfortunate* because large segments of the public have not always understood that the therapy was but one means of expressing the unifying principles as formulated by Andrew Taylor Still.

The philosophy of medicine proposed by Still was a unifying principle in itself and merited consideration in the practice of *all* phases of medicine. In every subdivision of internal medicine, surgery, and related medical specialties, the philosophy of medicine proposed by Still is applicable. It not only relates itself to manipulative therapy but it also provides a different perspective for the development of a more comprehensive system of medicine than had ever been realized before.

The individual principles that make up the philosophy of osteopathic medicine are being daily reaffirmed by contemporary osteopathic and medical re-

Today, in the five osteopathic colleges, anatomy is the foundation of an osteopathic education. An anatomy class at the Chicago College of Osteopathy is shown in this scene.

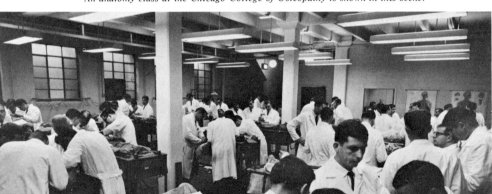

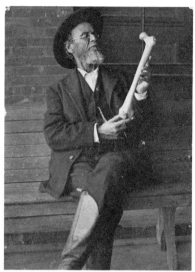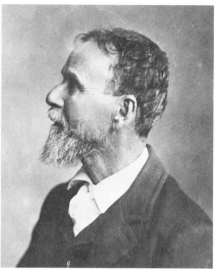

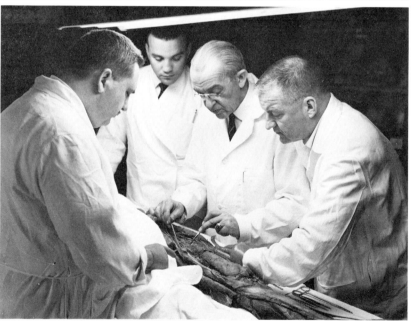

Top left: Still sought a basic philosophy in medicine soundly founded on anatomical and physiological principles. Top right: Andrew Taylor Still, 1828-1917, was both product and producer of nineteenth century Americana. Bottom: Formal education is a never-ending process for osteopathic physicians. Here Angus G. Cathie, D.O., works on a cadaver for the benefit of physicians taking a refresher course in anatomy given by the postgraduate division of the Philadelphia College of Osteopathy.

search. Yet the osteopathic profession is the sole system of medicine in the world today that has fully accepted and developed these basic philosophical principles as guidelines for practice and research into a better medicine for tomorrow. For example, the basic science of anatomy is taught in greater detail in osteopathic institutions than in any other medical educational centers. Osteopathic colleges are the only medical schools in the world that teach the functional changes that occur in the musculoskeletal system and instruct future physicians in a mechanical therapy for the relief of mechanical disorders to the body. And osteopathic medicine is the only profession which consistently teaches a pervading philosophy of body unity as it seeks to reveal the mysteries of health and the disasters of disease.

BODY UNITY

Body unity is more than a reasonable medical concept. It is a practical approach to health and disease. The need for such a practical application of this fundamental truth was recently pointed out by Nathan K. Rickles, M.D., chairman of the California State Mental Hygiene and Health Committee. Dr. Rickles wrote: "The medical school curriculum contains no adequate program to deal with the picture of the total man. Paradoxically, the very man who insists on detailed, exacting learning in the basic sciences apparently expects the unprepared student to absorb by osmosis the other related facts of life." The California physician continues: "The concept of the doctor treating the total man is a wholesome theme on which to base a doctor's education, but it requires amplification as well as implementation to be carried out effectively. Herein lies the crucial gap in our medical education today."

Thus it can be seen that although the importance of a study of man in his totality is recognized by individual old-school physicians, it is the osteopathic profession that makes a major issue of body unity in both its research and educational programs.

It is only when a physician begins to study a patient as a total biological unit —similar to all other such units in its gross aspects but differing from each in many important details—that the physician truly begins to approach the central focus of health and disease. Medicine must be more than an attempt to repair, relieve, or remove the end products of disease processes. A gallstone does not appear in a healthy gallbladder. Neither does the gallbladder become "sick" all by itself. Its nerve and blood supply and the chemical balance of body fluid must first be disturbed and in a state of disorder. The nervous system, the glandular system, and the circulatory system affect and are affected by reactions of the total body. To remove a gallbladder, diseased as it may be, does not represent a return of the body to a state of health. It is merely the removal of the debris of a disease yet undetected and untreated.

It is a known biological fact that when man is in a state of health he is healthy all over. Equally, when he is sick he is sick all over. The body is not a series of autocratic compartments bound together by the skin and skeletal system. It is not a biological apartment house with separate floors and no intercommunicating doors. It is a commune—an interrelated group of body organs and systems sharing in the common rights and property of a biological community.

THEORY IS MODERN

The theory of body unity or the interrelation of body functions is not contrary to the concepts of individual modern medical philosophers and scientists. Professor René Dubos of New York City's Rockefeller Institute, in discussing germs as a "cause" of disease, describes it this way: "The belief that disease can be conquered through the use of drugs deserves special attention here because it is widely held. Its fallacy is that it fails to take into account the difficulties arising on the ecological complexity of human problems. Blind faith in drugs is an attitude comparable to the naive cowboy philosophy that permeates the wild west thriller. In the crime-ridden frontier town the hero single-handedly blasts out the desperadoes who have been running rampant through the settlement. The story ends on a happy note because it appears that peace has been restored. But in reality the death of the villain does not solve the fundamental problem, for the rotten social conditions which opened the town to the desperadoes would soon allow others to come in unless something is done to correct the primary source of the trouble. The hero moves out of town without doing anything to solve this far more complex problem: in fact, he has no weapon to deal with it and is not even aware of its existence. Similarly, the accounts of miraculous cures rarely make clear that arresting an acute episode does not solve the problem of disease in the social body—or even in the individual concerned."

REMOVAL NOT ANSWER

The removal of a diseased gallbladder or the use of an antibiotic to combat germs that cause disease is a valuable and acceptable practice of osteopathic

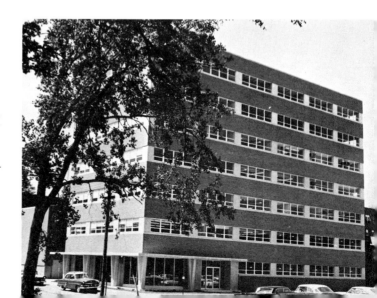

Research in support of osteopathic concepts has come a long way since the beginnings of the American system of medicine founded in the previous century. Keeping in step with the need for modern facilities, the Kirksville College of Osteopathy and Surgery recently completed this new Research Building.

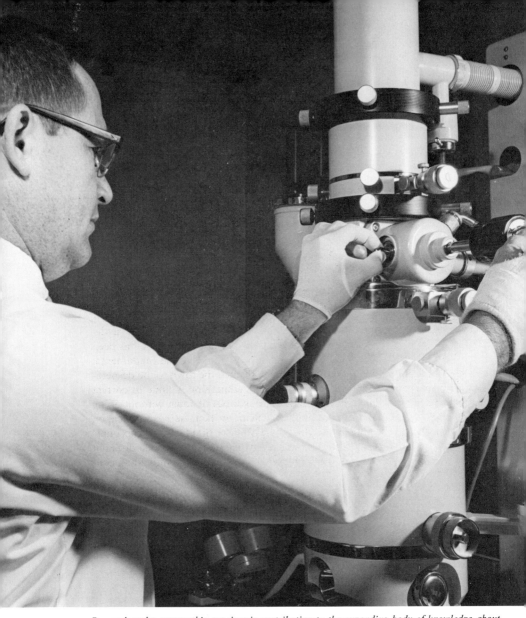

Research under osteopathic auspices is contributing to the expanding body of knowledge about the anatomy, physiology, and chemistry of the human body. In this scene, a neurophysiologist on the faculty of the College of Osteopathic Medicine and Surgery, Des Moines, Iowa, inserts a tissue specimen in the electron microscope for study. (*Lynn Baldwin*).

physicians. However, osteopathic medicine does not believe that the removal of diseased organs or the shooting of "desperado" germs with magic antibiotic bullets rids the biological community of total man of disease or constitutes the sole answer to man's health problems. It does little to rid the body of the poor environmental conditions within and without that permitted the disease to grow in the first place. Like the "crime-ridden town" of Dubos' allegory, the fundamental errors that were there in the first place still persist. The integration of these principles, particularly the one on body unity, too rarely enters the "practical" practice of medicine. If the philosophy is worthy of acceptance, the philosophy is worthy of practice.

A tubercle bacillus, by itself, is not tuberculosis. Neither is a tubercle bacillus that is placed in man tuberculosis. Medical science reveals that most of us who have reached maturity show evidence of invasion of the tubercle bacillus and its successful repulsion. This was accomplished not by the lungs, not by the musculoskeletal system, nor by any single system of the body. It was accomplished by the interaction of all of the forces of man in health providing an environment inconsistent with the development of disease. It is the contention of osteopathic medicine that, in the maintenance of health and the treatment of disease, a consideration of body unity has an important place in the diagnosis and treatment of the diseased condition.

INTERRELATED SYSTEMS

The unifying forces in the body are the nervous and circulatory systems. Every cell of the body is directly or indirectly under the influence of the function of the brain and spinal nerves. Even the circulatory system with its vascular pump, the heart, and the miles of tubing that make up the blood vessels are usually subservient to the modifying control of the central nervous system.

The skull and spine are part of nature's protective covering for this vital system of the body. The spinal nerves emerge from between the segments of the spine in specially constructed sheaths and are transmitted all over the body. The interconnections and interactions of these nerves with each other challenge the imagination of the most modern and skilled electronic engineer. Anything causing abnormal irritation to these nerves can and does affect widespread body function. Because these nerves cross between joints and through muscles and are also responsible for their function, any abnormal alteration in the function of the musculoskeletal system can cause aberrations in the normal and healthy unity of the body. When this balanced interrelation of body systems is disturbed in any manner, disease processes are prone to develop. Thus it can be seen that Dr. Still's insistence that the musculoskeletal system and its disorders be considered an integral part in the maintenance of body unity and balance is founded upon sound scientific fact. And it is the contention of osteopathic medicine that such a philosophy is practical in its application to the maintenance of health and the treatment of disease and that a consideration of total man has an important place in the diagnosis and treatment of disease states.

The principle of body unity in human biology is one of the major scientific reasons why the osteopathic profession exists as a vocal minority in the world of medicine. The philosophy is accepted but its application is not widely practiced. The fact that such practice and integration into the more practical and applicable approaches to diagnosis and treatment are lacking constitutes a void in medicine that must be filled. It is an integral portion of osteopathic medicine's plan for a comprehensive medical reformation.

The unity of the body is but one part of this dynamic philosophy of osteopathic medicine. And it is of vital importance to the future development of "scientific" medicine.

In the tradition of A. T. Still, osteopathic physicians return to the study of the body in their approach to keeping man in a state of wellness. Here, Elliott L. Hix, Ph.D., of the Kirksville College of Osteopathy and Surgery, lectures at a state osteopathic meeting. (Len Heffel).

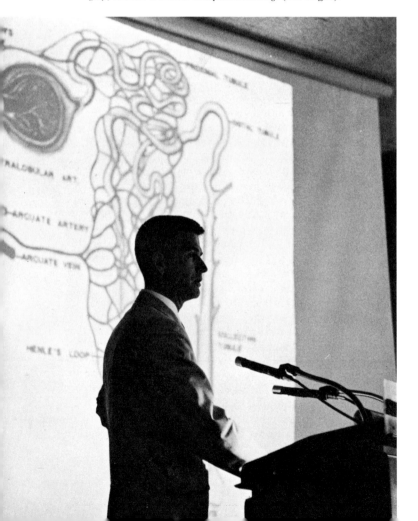

IV

VIS MEDICATRIX
NATURAE

The healing power of nature, *vis medicatrix naturae,* has always been a natural phenomenon of man. Since ancient times, the power of the body to maintain health and combat disease has been one of the fundamental ideas of medicine.

As a basic principle of osteopathic medicine, in both theory and practice, the body's tendency toward health and antipathy to disease is a fundamental condition for diagnosis and treatment. Order and health are universally one, in union. Disorder and disease are equally synonymous. Osteopathic medicine's founder, Andrew Taylor Still, described it thus: "We say disease when we should say effect; for disease is the effect of a change in the parts of the physical body. Disease in an abnormal body is just as natural as is health when all parts are in place."

Dr. Still did more than reaffirm "the healing force of nature." The significance of this dictum to osteopathic medicine was not its recognition but rather its practical application to the maintenance of health in the treatment of disease.

The concept that the body has within it those forces and chemicals necessary for the maintenance of health and the struggle against disease is a principle of major proportion for the practice of medicine. The body's internal and external environments must maintain an adaptable balance and unity. It is the ability of the body of fluctuate and meet various forms of stresses adequately and without exaggeration that proclaims a state of health. But when disorder within the body disrupts its healthful adaptability, or when man's external environment overcomes the checks and balances of body function, disease supervenes.

Congenital defects in body structure and function are commonly recognized disorders of internal body unity. Anatomic and metabolic (chemical) inherited abnormalities condition the body toward disease.

Fortunately, major congenital defects are not as common as one might believe.

EACH IS DISTINCT

Despite the comparative rarity of gross mechanical defects, every individual possesses a distinctively individual anatomic construction. The familiar observation that no two fingerprints are identical may be extended to more complex body structures. It could be said with equal truth that no two stomachs are identical, no two nervous systems are capable of the same responses, and no two brains contain duplicate storehouses of experience and information. Yet all of these "structures" respond through function. And the structure is inseparably welded to the function. Thus, despite the gross similarities of all men and all women, each person responds to internal and external situations in a fashion that typifies his own individuality. Construing further, it can be seen that every individual possesses his own capacity for health, which results in his own, personalized resistance to disease. The individuality of man is an important consideration for those who would understand man's nature.

Despite these individual variations, the human body responds to a variety of stressful situations with remarkable constancy. In fact, the ability of the body to adapt itself to environmental changes is the essence of health.

The external environment of man, however, is constantly overloading the body's tolerance for stress. Many of these stressful situations are willfully produced by the foolishness of man himself: drug addiction, food addiction, tobacco addiction, and other forms of psychophysical excesses all impinge upon nature and her tendencies toward health and away from disease.

The healing power of nature manifests itself daily. The knitting of bones in a fracture, the healing of a cut, the "wall" built around an infection as in a boil are all examples of the body's attempt to heal itself. Any treatment regime should be supportive of that attempt providing the compensatory mechanisms of the body to combat disease do not themselves become a source of irritation.

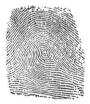

Like fingerprints, which are unique to the person who bears them, the structure of man's components and their over-all configuration are distinctly individual. No two of us are identical: one of the results is that no two persons have the same resistance to disease.

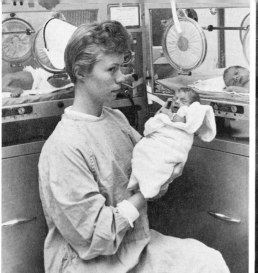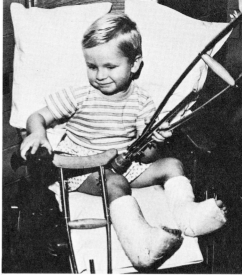

Left: These triplets, born at the Hospital of Philadelphia College of Osteopathy, weigh only about four pounds each. Thus, they are placed in incubators to provide a better environment for their growth. The intent of all treatment should be to support, stimulate, and sometimes initiate the natural predilection for health. (Philadelphia Inquirer). Right: The knitting together of broken bones—in fact, one's agonized attempt to hold an injured limb still, affording a natural splint to speed healing—represent the body's ordinary attraction for the healthy state. (National Society for Crippled Children and Adults, Inc.).

BODY COMPENSATES

The ability of the body to compensate for malevolent stresses, both internal and external, is protean. Compensation for disorder may be adequate, but it never constitutes normalcy. It is, however, a manifestation of the natural tendency of the body toward health when disturbed by disease, and the art of healing could not exist without it. The healing power of nature constitutes a powerful and vital resistance toward disordered unity. Treatment directed to the living body is meaningless except as an appeal to such powers of resistance as a patient possesses. As J. M. Dorsey, M.D., recently wrote in *The Journal of the Michigan State Medical Society,* "The human system is the only possible system of therapeutics (treatment)."

Disease therefore becomes a struggle for health within the economy of man's nature. William Harvey (1578-1657), the discoverer of the circulation of the blood, also wisely proclaimed, "Nature herself must be our advisor; the path she walks must be our walk." To neglect the *vis medicatrix naturae* is to neglect the manpower needed for recovery. The things that we recognize as being manifestations of disease, the so-called pathological findings, are really recognizable as drastic therapeutic efforts of the body's tissue—the body acting on its own initiative to secure relief.

STATE OF EQUILIBRIUM

Over 2,500 years ago, Alkmaion described health "as a state of equilibrium of the bodily powers or functions." This important equilibrium that maintains a

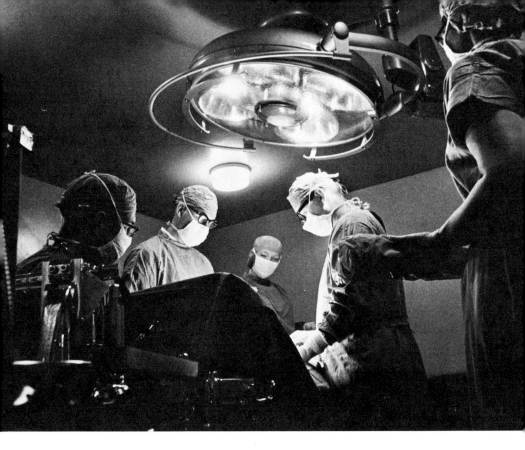

Repair, removal, or relief—the three R's of medicine—do not mark the zenith of achievement by physicians. Safeguarding health and preventing disease, which osteopathic medicine stresses, are higher goals. (Davenport, Iowa, Osteopathic Hospital).

successful struggle for health must become a practical and applicable basis for the practice of medicine.

Osteopathic medicine's founder, Andrew Taylor Still, continually "fought against the traditional ignorance of the power of nature to cure both old and young." This ignorance is not as prevalent in the practice of modern medicine as it was in the time of Still. The application of the fact, however, is far too frequently ignored because of the lack of a pervading philosophy for the practice of medicine. It is the contention of osteopathic medicine that there should be a broad basic philosophy upon which to build a more scientific and rational health practice and a higher order in the recognition and treatment of disease. The natural tendencies of the body toward health and its built-in mechanisms to combat disease make possible the art of healing. Without the propensity of the body to develop this power and vital resistance to disease, the art of healing would be impossible.

Unfortunately, medicine has not always placed as great an importance on the nature of health as it has on the nature of disease. A Stanford University pathologist, Lelland Joseph Rather, M.D., speaking before the International

Congress for Logic, Methodology and Philosophy of Science, said it in this manner: "If we measure interest by activities rather than by protestations, physicians have been and are, for the most part, as little interested in health as soldiers in peace." The validity of this statement and the fundamental truths expressed in the concept of *"vis medicatrix naturae"* make vitally necessary a continuing reformation in the practice of medicine as we know it. Dr. Still admonished the physicians of osteopathic medicine, "To find health should be the object of the doctor." In modern times, Rockefeller Institute's René DuBos said, "Most of the disorders of the body and the mind are but the expressions of inadequate responses to environmental influences." These are not the mouthings of armchair philosophers but rather the "voices in the wilderness" that are students of man's very nature.

NATURE'S POWER

The areas of medical science where the healing power of nature has been both recognized and used have been most productive. The fact that this natural phenomenon is not a practiced philosophy throughout all phases of medicine is self-evident. There is, however, one shining example of its use—in the field of preventive medicine, particularly as it relates to the immunization of large sections of our population against infectious diseases. The immunization procedure depends solely on its ability to support and stimulate man's resistance against "specific" infections. Smallpox, diphtheria, whooping cough, tetanus, and, particularly in our time, poliomyelitis are outstanding examples of the practical application of the natural ability of the body, when properly stimulated, to manufacture within itself those elements necessary to resist disease. The future of medicine will reveal that there are other aspects of body health that can be maintained and stimulated through appropriate measures.

The body's response to gravity and ability to maintain a balanced upright position are rarely discussed when one considers the healing power of nature. Yet, man is a mechanical being, subject to mechanical stresses and strains, and

The founder of osteopathy declared that the doctor should purpose to find health. Preventive medicine exemplifies this resolve. Here, influenza virus is harvested for vaccine. (Eli Lilly and Co.).

is constantly struggling to maintain his positional balance and overcome the forces of gravity, which are literally trying to drive him into the ground.

ARCHITECTURAL MASTERPIECE

The normal structure, with its parts of the body in proper relationship, one to the other, is an architectural masterpiece for the preservation of balance and mobility against gravity's force. When that balance is disturbed by mechanical distortion, however, balance disappears and unbalance is a result. The normal anatomy of the body, which provides agility and mobility, is distorted when distortion appears in structure. Therefore, the ability of the body to compensate for abnormal mechanical stresses and strains is an important factor in the study of man and his normal healing capacities. The inter-relationship of anatomic parts and their dependency on one another are major considerations in any study of body dysfunction or disease.

The recognition of the mechanical factor of *vis medicatrix naturae* is distinctively osteopathic in its concept. Until the advent of osteopathic medicine, it was a missing link in the study of man.

Basically, *all* treatment should be designed to support, stimulate, and in some instances initiate the body's trend toward health. The three R's of medicine— repair, remove, and relieve—are not sufficient unto themselves. Relief, removal, or repair is necessary and helpful but is primarily designed to cope with the by-products of disease rather than with the disease itself. It is in the field of prevention and the support of health that osteopathic medicine maintains an emphasis.

TOTALITY, UNITY

The concept of body unity is inseparable from any consideration of the natural healing capacity of man. No system of the body, including the musculoskeletal system, can be left out when considering the totality and the unity of the body. It likewise follows any consideration of the healing power of the body must also be all-inclusive. Without such consideration, a truly comprehensive system of medicine can never be achieved.

Medicine, today, needs a pervading philosophical base upon which to build. Cornerstones for that base must include both the body's unity and its natural healing capacities. The recognition of the healing power of the body is common to physicians of all ages. Its emphasis and applications as basic formulations for a needed philosophy of medicine is uniquely emphasized in the principles of osteopathic medicine.

These principles have ancient origin, modern applications, and promises of new discoveries that augur well for the establishment of a system of comprehensive medicine unrealized in our time. It is toward such a reformation that the osteopathic profession moves from the flexibility of its minority position to a more stable and fundamentally sound medical practice for tomorrow.

V

THE MECHANICAL FACTOR IN HEALTH AND DISEASE

"Functional" has become a favorite twentieth-century adjective. Individuals and organizations desire to be functional. There are functional furniture, functional architecture, and even functional medicine.

Function, however, presupposes a structure that makes it possible: structure determines function, and function is a modifier of structure. Structure and function are inseparable in both inanimate and animate forms. Thus, because of the intimate bond between the framework and the workings of the human body, the structure-function concept has been developed as a basic premise of osteopathic medicine.

THE SEED

Where does an idea start? As an "original" idea in the mind of one person? Hardly so. The origin of an idea is rarely certain, and too much energy often is expended in fixing the credit, which more often than not goes to the one who first puts the idea to good use. Therefore, the idea of the reciprocal relationship between structure and function has been attributed to Dr. Andrew Taylor Still, the founder of osteopathy, because he was one of the first to make practical application of this fundamental concept in the diagnostics and therapeutics of medicine. Whether Dr. Still has received more or less credit for the structure-function concept than he deserves is of minor importance. It is, however, of major importance that he recognized the validity of the concept and applied it in diagnosis and therapy.

There is historical evidence that the biological marriage of structure to function was recognized as a fundamental idea early in medical history.

Rudolf Virchow (1821-1902), generally acclaimed as one of the greatest scientists of the nineteenth century, wrote in 1855 that "all diseases can be reduced to disturbances of the aberrant composition and *structure* of the molecules of the cell and hence to physically and chemically detectable changes as expressed by aberrant *function*." Yet, even today, it is only the occasional student of medicine who realizes the importance of the application of this principle to the practice of his profession.

GREAT MINDS

Dr. Still, probably unaware of Virchow's earlier statement, nevertheless set forth ideas similar to this when he recognized and studied the inseparability of structure and function in man. There is an interesting comparison between the approaches toward truth made by Virchow and Still. Virchow was a pathologist, a student of the debris of disease. He was a student of the structure-function of body disorder and disharmony in death, whereas Still was a student primarily of the anatomy and physiology of life. They traveled along different perimeters but arrived at similar conclusions. Such is the nature of truth.

Thus, prior to Dr. Still's observations and conclusions, Virchow had formulated the structure-function theory at the molecular level of the cell. Prior to Virchow's time, however, the great German scientist Theodor Schwann (1810-1882) had made similar observations concerning the cell as a total unit. What Still had declared as being a biological truth in its grosser aspect — namely, that the anatomy of the body is an important factor in determining its physiology—Schwann and Virchow were hypothesizing at the cellular and molecular levels. One was the observation of gross structure-function changes and the other of microscopic ones. The basic truth was the same, however, and the facts remain incontrovertible.

"Virchow and Cellular Pathology" (©*1961, Parke, Davis & Company)—In 1855, Dr. Rudolf Virchow, while professor at Wurzburg University, Germany, set forth his theory that disease results from disturbances in cells by injury or irritants.*

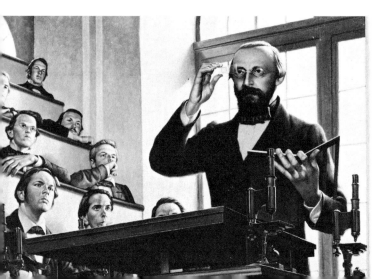

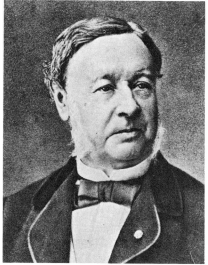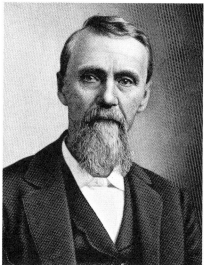

Left: Theodor Schwann (1810-1882), German professor of anatomy and physiology, is credited with the development of cellular theory. (Bettmann Archive). Right: Although Dr. Still was probably unaware of Virchow's cell-disturbance theory, he expounded similar ideas in recognizing and studying the inseparability of structure and function in man.

New information on the structure-function concept did not cease to flow in the nineteeth century. With the advent of the twentieth century and the launching of the atomic age, the importance of the structure-function concept was recognized to include the atomic level.

It was in 1919 that the first nuclear reaction took place. Then, on December 2, 1942, at the University of Chicago, the first controlled atomic fission, or "atomic splitting," was accomplished. And now, subatomic structure-function considerations are under investigation.

A PRINCIPLE TENET

The structure-function concept has always been a cornerstone of osteopathic principle and practice. A great student of human anatomy, Dr. Still noted that abnormalities occurring in the anatomical *structure* of the body resulted in abnormal *function*. Although he was observing alterations primarily in the gross structure of the musculoskeletal system, Dr. Still realized that, not only was the function of the muscle-ligament-bone complex altered, but that functional disturbances were occurring in the closely related nervous and circulatory systems as well.

This fundamental—the sensitive interdependence that exists between structure and function—if given proper development, may set in motion a total reformation of medical thought.

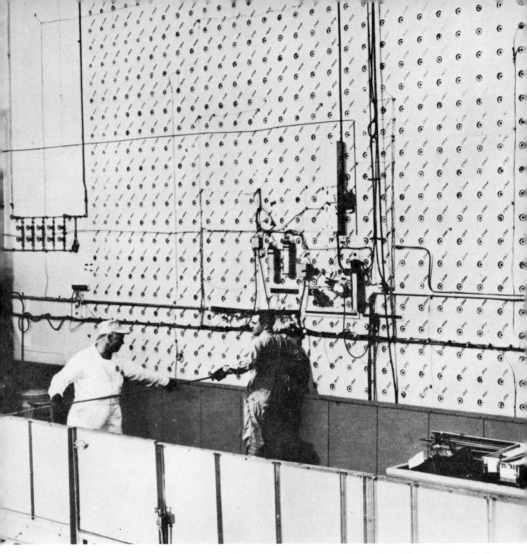

This is the Oak Ridge (Tenn.) nuclear reactor. Substances to be irradiated for isotope production are encased and placed in the holes shown. After weeks or months they become radioactive and are removed for processing. (Abbott Laboratories).

MANIPULATION REBORN

It was from the studies of Still that the rediscovery of a long-neglected treatment aid—manipulative therapy—was intensively developed by the osteopathic profession. If osteopathic medicine were no more and no less than the only medical educational system that teaches this logical diagnostic and therapeutic approach to the problems of health and disease, the profession would nonetheless be making a contribution of major proportions.

With Still's application of the structure-function concept to the study of health and disease in man, a new and practical recognition was achieved. One educator has referred to it as the recognition of "mechanical man." The chemical, the mental, and the spiritual aspects of man's nature had long been recognized, but very little attention had been paid to the structural-functional mechanics of the human body. Even today, osteopathic institutions represent the only system of medical education presenting these views for the usefulness of its practitioners. Colleges of osteopathic medicine are the *only* medical centers in the world where structural body diagnosis and manipulative techniques are taught as an integral, inseparable part of the medical curriculum.

The recognition that man can become mechanically disordered and that this in turn can adversely affect the body's normal trend to health is a cardinal and distinctive contribution of osteopathic medicine. It is a critical consideration and should become a part of the teaching of every recognized medical school in the country. To fail to teach this basic principle of medicine and its appendant diagnostic and therapeutic methods is to prepare incompletely a physician for public service. To gain better acceptance and understanding of the structure-function concept is one of the major objectives of the osteopathic profession. Further study of this concept must be continuous and exhaustive, for it augurs well to be a cornerstone of the medicine of the future.

UNIFYING PHILOSOPHY

It is to Still's credit that he was one of the first to make practical application of the structure-function concept. It can be seen that the concept has strong fundamental support, both historic and contemporary, as a basic idea for a philosophy of medicial practice.

No careful student of biological man can escape the validity of this approach. Whether one alters the gross structure of the body by manipulative therapy or whether one "manipulates" the molecular structure of a cell by radiation, chemicals, and means yet to be determined, the resulting altered function cannot be denied.

Thus, in the concepts of total body unity, the inherent predilection of the body for health, and its natural healing forces—combined with the broad implications manifest in the structure-function concept—osteopathic medicine has for the first time initiated the construction of a basic, unifying philosophy for the study of man, his health, his disease.

PREPARING THE WAY

The distinguished American physiologist Irvin M. Korr, Ph.D., chairman of the Division of Physiological Sciences of the Kirksville (Mo.) College of Osteopathy and Surgery, visualizes the fundamental principles of osteopathic medicine as providing the next higher stage of medicine through initiation and participation in a medical reformation.

Dr. Korr states: "The next stage of medicine will be one that better meets the health needs of the day and that better anticipates the rapidly changing needs of modern society. It will not be concerned only with the recognizing, preventing, and treating of individual episodes and types of illness; it will direct its primary efforts at the fullest exploitation, liberation and development of man's natural biological resources for productive life. It will be engaged much less in *intervening* in the inconceivably complex biological processes of the human organism than in creating circumstances, in and around the individual, that will *permit* their optimal operation and *eliminate impediments* to their operation."

"This emerging, higher stage of medicine will be concerned with the identification and control of those factors and variables in the individual, in the human organism as a species, in human life, and in society, and in the environment that significantly and decisively influence the ability to stay on optimal physiologic paths, to resist deflection from those paths, and to return to them. Its efforts will be directed not so much at the so-called specific causes of disease as at the factors that permit them to *become* causes. Its concern will be more with the elimination and control of factors contributing to susceptibility to illness in general than with the cataloging of diseases and their treatment in their endless variety. It will combat disease not so much by fragmented and expedient attempts on *diseases* as by concerted programs for maintenance and improvement of health—for 'raising levels of wellness.' "

Speaking at his office at the Timken Burnett Memorial Research Building of the Kirksville College, Dr. Korr recently reiterated his long-held belief: "I am deeply convinced that the next higher stage of medicine—long on the way and now desperately needed—will be guided by those principles which, in their continually evolving form, constitute the 'osteopathic concept.' "

At the root of this concept are the basic principles of osteopathic medicine. Surely one of the most signal of them is the consideration of structure-function and its relation to health and disease.

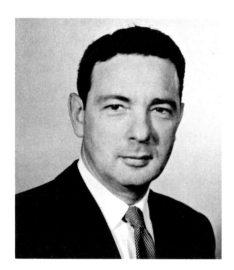

Irvin M. Korr, Ph.D., chairman of the Division of Physiological Sciences at the Kirksville College of Osteopathy and Surgery, predicts that the next stage of medicine will "combat disease not so much by fragmented and expedient attempts on diseases as by concerted programs for maintenance and improvement of health—for 'raising levels of wellness.' " Moreover, it will "be guided by those principles which, in their continually evolving form, constitute the 'osteopathic concept,' " he say.

VI

A MYSTERIOUS LESION

The musculoskeletal system comprises more than 60 per cent of the mass of the total body structure. In the study of the structure and function of man as interwoven, interdependent phenomena, the musculoskeletal system can no longer be considered as an anatomical hat rack that merely supports the "important" organs of the body. Other important tasks depend on this system, and, in fact, all parts of it—the bones, muscles, tendons, ligaments, and fascia—must be of the proper construction and relationship to work properly. A person needs only to sprain his ankle to realize this truth.

One of the major objectives of osteopathic medicine is to establish the musculoskeletal system in its proper perspective in the hierarchy of body systems. It is a system of importance unto itself and of importance, often unrecognized, to the proper function of other body parts. If the "whole-body concept" of osteopathic medicine is as valid as we believe it to be, certainly particular attention and emphasis should be directed to that system that constitutes 60 per cent of our being.

BIPEDALISM

From time immemorial, we have been lectured concerning proper posture. We are told to "stand straight," "pull in the stomach," and avoid the "debutante slouch." Too often we accept this time-honored advice as useful if convenient but fail to understand the important bearing that good posture has on total body health.

Man with all the glory of his unique upright posture has reaped many benefits. The mobility and agility of two-legged man have helped to maintain his dominance over the animal kingdom. (If you doubt this, try walking around on all fours for a few seconds.) Whether man originated as a two-legged creature or became one through evolutionary changes is relatively unimportant to this discussion; the fact that he is a biped *is* important. The upright position, however, carries with it both assets and handicaps.

The assets are obvious, the handicaps less clear. Upright man is engaged in a continual battle against the forces of gravity and the maintenance of equilibrium. Too often we conceive of the structure of the human body as a series of blocks supporting one's position in space. Too often also we think of the spinal column as a relatively immobile object moving only when we voluntarily command it to do so. Yet, medical science reveals that the body's structural components are rarely still: every time we inhale and exhale, the spine, the ribs, and the muscles attached thereto are in motion. No matter how minimal, motion is always present and persistent. The human respiratory rate is approximately 20 respirations per minute. Multiplying the minutes by the hours and the hours by the days and the days by the months and the months by the years—that's a lot of motion. Yet the structure of our bodies has so adapted to function that wear and tear are minimized.

Man, however, continually abuses his musculoskeletal system. Modern furniture, compact cars, and occupational hazards place stresses on "mechanical man" with which he was not designed to cope. Added to these environmental hazards is the additional impediment that people are creatures of habit. We have two legs, but we often stand with most of our weight on one. For sitting, we build our chairs with seats so long that if we were to place our back against

The osteopathic profession is laying the groundwork to meet the challenge of the growing need of more physicians to take care of the health needs of an exploding American population. All five of the osteopathic colleges have plans on drawing boards or are already in the process of building to expand its facilities to accommodate more students. In addition, a new college is being founded in Pontiac, Mich. The architect's model of the Michigan College of Osteopathic Medicine complex to be developed over a 20-year period is shown here.

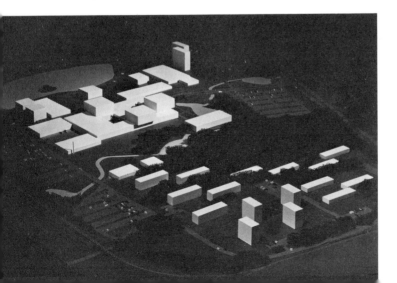

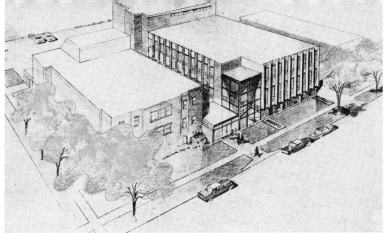

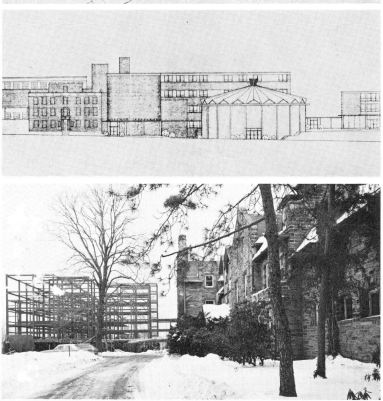

Top: Included in the first stage of a 10-year expansion program at the Chicago College of ʼeopathy is a new science building. The $10 million building expansion project also ʼes an addition to the present hospital, a new clinical laboratory and pathology ..ꞔꝑ.. ꞵꜩent, a new outpatient diagnostic and treatment clinic, and an additional hospital wing. Center: A new science-research building is one of the priority projects of the $10-million development program that is in progress at the Kansas City College of Osteopathy and Surgery. Bottom: The Philadelphia College of Osteopathy broke ground for its new $7.2 million hospital in mid-1965 and by winter had reached the construction stage shown here. The new hospital is going up on the College's City Line campus near the mansion that now houses the administration offices.

41

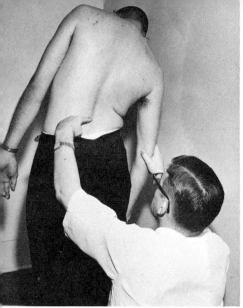
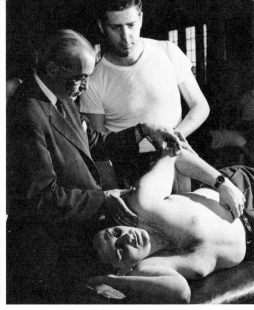

Left: Ira C. Rumney, D.O., professor of osteopathic theory and practice at the Kirksville College of Osteopathy and Surgery, looks for asymmetry in his patient during the physical examination. Right: Angus G. Cathie, D.O., professor of osteopathic principles and practice at the Philadelphia College of Osteopathy, pinpoints osteopathic lesion for a student.

the back of the chair our feet would be off the ground. Not wishing to assume such an undignified and uncomfortable position, we place our feet on the floor and literally warp our bodies into all sorts of peculiar and stressful positions. The habit of sitting cross-legged is also common practice, and we invariably get in the habit of sitting with the same leg crossed over the other. Man was designed to distribute his weight equally between the two halves of the body, but man has designed too often to do just the opposite. The result is constant and continuing strain to the body's framework.

As a result of the multitudinous strains to the structure-function works of the body, body symmetry is distorted. Changes in the normal musculoskeletal system occur, and disability results. Backaches, "bursitis," stiff necks, and other musculoskeletal complaints are legion. Man has been described facetiously as a "biped animal with a backache," an aphorism that bears too much truth.

Gross distortions of posture and the resultant loss of physical fitness have become popular considerations in our modern society. Courses of exercises and physical training have been proposed to counteract this threat to human comfort and efficiency. The late President John F. Kennedy's Council on Physical Fitness, carried forward and emphasized by President Lyndon B. Johnson, is a concrete example of the recognition of this growing problem.

With the assassination, President Kennedy's physical fitness program might have died as well, but with the appointment of baseball's great Stan Musial it is again occupying the spotlight. The American Osteopathic Association has cooperated with the President's Council on Physical Fitness in the production of a movie, "The Fitness Challenge," which has already been viewed by more than 3.5 million people.

MANIPULATIVE THERAPY

In the late 1800's the pioneer American physician Andrew Taylor Still recognized the importance of the musculoskeletal system in health and disease and its relation not only to itself but to other body systems. Through his study and research, he discovered that the joints of the body, particularly those of the spine, developed unusual manifestations of stress. He discovered that the effects of joint strains, transmitted through the nervous and circulatory systems, were not only local but often remote. He believed that their structure-function could be brought back toward normal by the use of manipulative therapy, which ancient treatment method he refined into a modern, precise therapeutic tool.

Originally, osteopathic physicians conceived that joint dysfunctions constituted minor subluxations (incomplete dislocations), the joint dysfunction being primarily a disturbance in function. They "reduced" them by carefully applied manipulations, and many cases responded spectacularly. These joint dysfunctions, however, have now been explored in greater depth with the development and research instituted by the osteopathic profession. Minor positional changes are but possible parts of the complete story.

OSTEOPATHIC LESIONS

A lesion is defined as a more-or-less circumscribed change in body tissue.

A common type of osteopathic lesion is similar to a sprain of tissues around any one of the body's joints. As a result, there is joint dysfunction, and motion is disturbed. The disturbance is usually a restriction of motion, and a joint so restricted is painful, since it is in constant use.

Every joint of the body is capable of voluntary motions. For example, the index finger can be bent forward and extended. These, however, are not all of the motions of which this joint is capable: there are accessory motions in a joint that are extremely important as well. By pulling on the end of the finger, the joint at the knuckle can be separated. By pushing the finger in, the surfaces of the joint come closer together. A certain amount of rotation can be made to occur in this joint, and gaping of the joint on either side may be accomplished. These accessory motions cannot be done voluntarily but can occur as a result of outside forces.

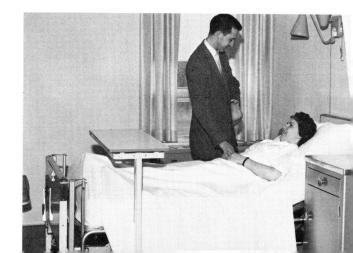

William G. McDowell, D.O., Sharon, Pa., general practitioner, checks up on his patient in Shenango Valley Osteopathic Hospital. More osteopathic physicians are G.P.s., or family doctors, than specialists.

It is these accessory motions of joints, not under direct voluntary control, that permit the normal "play" in joints. If these are impeded or lost, the joint no longer responds normally to the various stresses and strains imposed upon it. Because of the the lack of joint "give," normal motion becomes a source of irritation, and the irritation, in turn, causes tissue changes and swelling with resulting pain and nerve irritation. This series of events, in fact, constitutes an inflammatory reaction and can occur around various joints in the body, particularly the spine. Such a reaction is what the osteopathic profession generally refers to as an osteopathic lesion.

This series of changes is that originally described by Dr. Still when he was making his early investigations into the musculoskeletal system of the body. Time and study have broadened the original concept in importance and extensiveness. An osteopathic lesion may *sometimes* be a minor subluxation, but there are many other types.

One cannot precisely define an osteopathic lesion because mere words cannot adequately describe a whole body of observations. Recent study has indicated that these lesions may exist in several parts of the musculoskeletal system and that disturbances in one area create disorder in other areas. The osteopathic lesion cannot be demonstrated at autopsy for it is a *lesion of motion;* it is a disturbance in man's ability to adapt himself to the "normal" mechanical stresses of life.

SYSTEMS CLOSELY KNIT

The osteopathic lesion is much more than an occasional subluxation of a joint and much more than a response to mechanical trauma and stress. The musculoskeletal system is intimately connected with all other systems of the body through both the voluntary and the involuntary nervous systems. It is highly susceptible to changes in glandular function, and glandular function is itself so minutely connected with the nervous system that the two are often considered together as the neuroendocrine system.

Thus, indications are that the musculoskeletal system is a mirror of both health and disease, responding as it does to inflammation and pain from disorder in other body systems. An example of this response is the rigidity observed in the muscle over the right side of the abdomen when the appendix is inflamed: the muscle involuntarily contracts and is rigid and painful to the touch.

Similarly, other diseases cause disturbances in the musculoskeletal system and may in turn cause an osteopathic lesion. Recent studies have indicated that stomach ulcers consistently cause areas of spinal pain and irritation just below the shoulders in the back. The radiation of pain to the right shoulder from a diseased gallbladder is another typical example, and the reflection of pain and disability to the left shoulder following heart disease is a classic example. The important part in diagnosing such disorders lies in recognizing that symptoms can be produced without actual disorder in organs to which pain has been referred. Pain of spinal origin can mimic all of these diseases and, unless recog-

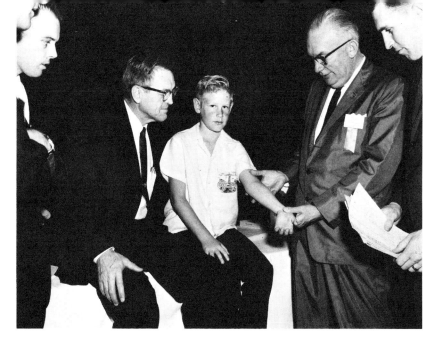

F. Munro Purse, D.O. (second from right), Narberth, Pa., a pediatrician, examines a youngster at the National Osteopathic Child Health Conference and Clinic in Kansas City, Mo. Myron D. Jones, D.O. (left), KCCOS professor of practice (pediatrics), and students watch.

nized, can have dangerous consequences. The osteopathic lesion is an important fact in medical diagnosis and treatment.

The concept of an osteopathic lesion as being solely a "bone out of place" must be abandoned owing to the force of facts. As pointed out, the musculo-skeletal system is not static; it is literally in constant motion. And the osteo-pathic lesion is a change in normal joint motion. Thus, it can only be observed in life and cannot be demonstrated in death. Likewise, it cannot be identified by static x-ray studies but will be more clearly viewed when "motion-picture x-rays" have been safely developed.

The osteopathic lesion is commonly missed as a diagnosis. There has been general acceptance of its role in such common things as low-back pain and various types of neuralgias. It is now more frequently being recognized as an imitator of other diseases. The pain typical of kidney stones may be identi-cally reproduced by disorders of function in the spine—yet another instance of one system's responding to another's ills.

MYSTERIOUS ROLE

The greatest importance of the osteopathic lesion may well lie in its potential relationship to the function of other body systems. This is perhaps its least understood and most mysterious quality. What *is* its role in the production of disorder, disharmony, and disease through its effect on the nervous system and hence its effect on the rest of the body? It is this particular facet of osteopathic medicine that is most challenging and requires the greatest research effort.

The osteopathic lesion, though only partially understood, has been demonstrated repeatedly in the offices of osteopathic physicians for almost a hundred years, and millions of patients have benefited from its recognition and treatment. Nonetheless, the osteopathic lesion's importance in degenerative diseases and so-called functional diseases and its relationship to total health must be better explained. To this end, the osteopathic profession maintains its institutions and organizations. As incomplete as our knowledge is, our several osteopathic colleges are the *only* medical institutions in the world that are teaching these concepts and investigating their potentiality.

The discoverable part of the mystery of the osteopathic lesion is the fact that it frequently occurs and that it may be readily recognized by trained osteopathic physicians through palpation (touch), a careful patient history, and a profound knowledge of anatomy and physiology. The unknown quality is an explanation of the many observations made relative to the osteopathic lesion by thousands of physicians over the past many years.

What *is* known is sufficient to provide the osteopathic physician with knowledge that greatly enhances his ability to diagnose disease and with added methods of treatment in which osteopathic physicians are proficient. Thus, this profession is able to furnish now a more comprehensive type of medical care than has ever been known. Combining the osteopathic body of knowledge with the other advancements in medicine and placing these concepts in their proper perspective is a contribution to the health care of all. It is a distinctive contribution for the benefit of *all* of medicine.

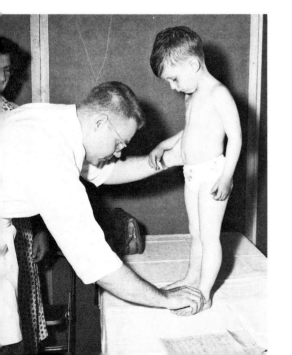

Thomas R. Turner, D.O., an orthopedic surgeon, examines a child's structure during the annual Fort Worth (Texas) Child Health Clinic, sponsored by the osteopathic profession.

VII

A PHYSICIAN
AND HIS HANDS

A group of East African natives had traveled far to obtain medical care. To the amazement of bystanders, the litter bearers carried the sick one past the doors of a large, imposing government hospital, continuing their journey until they reached a less pretentious hospital maintained by a mission station. When asked why they had walked the extra miles to the mission hospital, they replied in a strange manner: "The medicine may be the same, but the hands are different."

The care rendered by the mission doctors evidently communicated a compassion and understanding that took precedence over a shorter route and more attractive facilities. These humble people instinctively sought the art as well as the science of healing.

Millions of people throughout the world have sought the care of osteopathic physicians because "their hands are different." This is not to say that many physicians, M.D. and D.O., do not have unusual compassion for their patients. The crux of the difference, instead, is that the hands of osteopathic physicians have been schooled in techniques and methods of treatment not included in any other form of medical training.

Traditionally, the physician's hands have demonstrated his warmth and skill. The hands of the diagnostician explore the body, seeking the clues of disease. The hands of the surgeon, trained to precision performance, skillfully reconstruct or sometimes remove diseased organs. The handshake, the pat on the back, and the comforting pressure of a sympathetic hand convey more than words—a care for human life and dignity.

Since the beginning of recorded time, the hands of doctors have played a leading role in medical practice, and the use of massage in the treatment of the ill is recorded in earliest medical history. It seems an inborn trait of intelligent life to rub or massage accessible parts of the body that are bothersome: an aching muscle is massaged, a cramp is grasped, a tickling area is rubbed. Such responses are instinctive.

From ancient medicine, various forms of massage were carried into modern times as a part of medical care. It is reported that the oldest mention of massage is found in the Chinese *Kong-Fou* written about 2700 B.C. Massage was popular in the heyday of Greek and Roman life and became an integral part of early medical care. The Greek physician Aietaeus (first century A.D.) used it for the treatment of headache, vertigo, epilepsy, etc. The sanctuaries of Aesculapius promoted the use of massage by the priests plus the addition of magic incantations and suggestions.

Massage was practiced by slaves, priests, and physicians; Julius Caesar, Cicero, and Pliny were devotees of this form of therapy. In fact, throughout history famous people, both medical and nonmedical, have attested to its value.

Early contemporary interest in this therapy was particularly stirred with the establishment in 1813 by Pehr Henrik Ling of an institute of medical gymnastics in Stockholm. Calling his idea "kinestherapy," he developed a system of Swedish massage that won international fame.

Perhaps the greatest nineteenth century influence was that of Johann George Metzger, M.D., of Bonn. He instructed physicians in massage techniques and was known all over the world for the clinical results he was able to achieve. Typical of the respect with which he was held, a newspaper cartoon of the time pictured Bismarck talking to Metzger and saying, "I believed I had power in my hands, but I can see you have Europe's rulers under your thumb."

Therefore since the time of Galen, who was said to have written 16 books

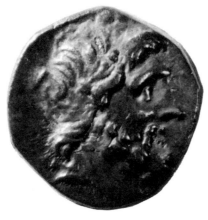

"Head of Asklepios." This portrait is on a silver drachma, a Greek coin minted on the island of Cos, dated about 150 B.C. The commonest version of the origin of this legendary figure—the Greek god of medicine, called Aesculapius by the Romans—is that he was the son of Apollo. (*Philadelphia Museum of Art*).

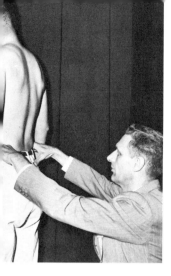

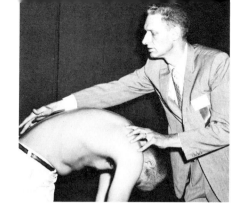

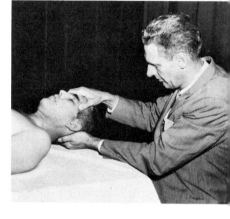

Osteopathic physicians rely on what they feel with their hands in conducting a structural examination. In these three pictures, Paul E. Kimberly, D.O., of St. Petersburg, Fla., demonstrates some of the things he looks for during an examination. Above, he kneels to determine the height of the ilium. Above right, he has the patient bend forward to check the level of the sacrum. Right, cervical motion is checked.

on exercise and massage, some form of manipulative therapy has been considered beneficial in the maintenance of health and the prevention and treatment of disease.

With progress, another early form of manual treatment grew in popularity: the reposition of broken and dislocated bones. And, sporadically throughout medical history, occasional observers have noted the benefits of manipulation as applied to body joints in the alleviation of both local joint pain and remote disturbances, caused by the irritation of branches of nerves in proximity to the disturbed joint.

Nevertheless, it was not until the advent of Andrew Taylor Still, founder of osteopathic medicine, that manipulative therapy was placed on a rational basis. It has been through the development of the osteopathic profession, its colleges and hospitals, and its research programs that the diagnostic importance of joint dysfunction to the total health of the body has been realized.

EARLY ENGLISH MANIPULATORS

Prior to the time of Dr. Still, particularly in England, the "bonesetter" flourished with increasing success. Though often skilled, many of these early bonesetters,

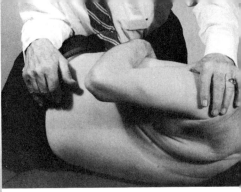

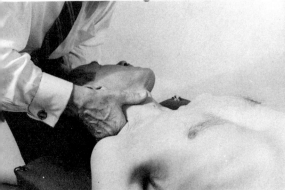

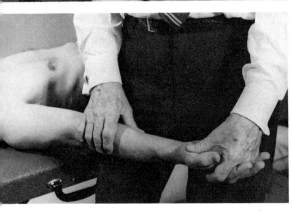

*The normalization of the disturbed
structure-function of the joints and
supporting tissues is what the osteopathic physician works toward in
applying manipulative treatment
whether it involves the neck area,
shoulder, the extremities, or any other
part of the body.*

unfortunately, had no formal medical training. Despite this lack, the first
English doctor to receive the high honor of a baronetcy, Sir Hans Sloane of
the College of Physicians, turned to the notorious bonesetter Mrs. Mapp to
have his niece cured of a spinal deformity. It was said of this early eighteenth-
century practitioner-of-sorts that "Dame nature has given her a doctor's degree— she gets all your patients and pockets the fee."

In 1867, the distinguished English physician Sir James Paget warned his
medical colleagues: "Few of you are likely to practice without having a bonesetter for a rival; and if he can cure a case which you have failed to cure, his
fortune may be made and yours marred." Although Paget was highly skeptical
of many of the claims made for the cures, he pointed out that the bonesetter
who had performed the cure might live on it for the rest of his life, whereas
the physician who failed to recognize the benefits and skills of the method
was the one whose reputation suffered.

Perhaps it is Sir James Paget's admonition that has caused the recent development in England of the Association of Manipulative Medicine, whose

membership is composed entirely of M.D.s. However, the fact of the matter is that in North America medical leaders and educators have almost completely failed to recognize the need for this training by all physicians who care for the sick. At the present time, such training is only available in the five osteopathic colleges. It should be a part of the complete training of a physician, and for this reason osteopathic medicine teaches a distinctive diagnostic technique and therapy *as a part* of a total and complete medical education. Thus, the comprehensiveness of osteopathic medicine is achieved.

NO MASSAGE

When the final page of medical history is written, it will be said that it was Dr. Still and osteopathic medicine that achieved the general recognition of the value of manipulation in the treatment of many and diverse conditions.

Osteopathic manipulative therapy is far more than massage: it is based upon specific diagnosis, indicated or contra-indicated by the individual requirements of the patient, and scientifically applied through the training and experience of skilled osteopathic physicians.

Despite vigorous opposition, particularly notable in the early days of the osteopathic profession's development, the fact of structural malfunction of joints and related muscles, ligaments, and musculoskeletal connecting tissue has received a growing acceptance by all of medicine. This is particularly true in the acknowledgment of local joint dysfunction. Manipulative treatment is gradually assuming its proper place in the management of low back pain due to mechanical disorder, stiff and painful necks and shoulders, and various types of pains referred to other areas of the body from joint disturbances.

Nonetheless, even though the diagnostic technique be important and the manipulator skilled, manipulative therapy must be predicated upon a sound and general knowledge of all of medicine. This the osteopathic physician has by dint of his training. Completely trained in all phases of internal medicine, obstetrics, and surgery, the osteopathic physician brings a form of comprehensive medical care to the advantage of his patient that other practitioners do not.

An intern visits with a patient as he makes his rounds at the Davenport (Iowa) Osteopathic Hospital.

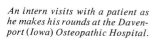

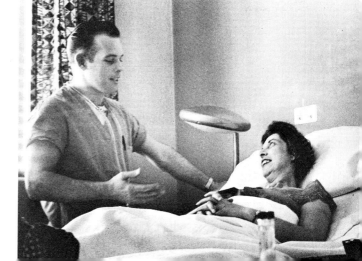

Come with me into the office of a contemporary osteopathic physician. Sitting opposite his consultation desk is the perennially typical patient "Mrs. Jones." This morning she bent over to pick up her young child, felt "something give" in her back, and could not straighten up without excruciating pain. She is now in pain and also fearing the worst. She has learned, however, to have confidence in her osteopathic physician because he has seen her husband through a mild heart attack, has delivered her babies and immunized her children against the childhood diseases, and is known in his community as an understanding and skilled physician.

Mrs. Jones thinks she has a "bone out of place" and needs manipulative treatment, but she does not know what actually has happened and neither does the osteopathic physician—until he has completed a careful history and physical examination. Although the D.O. is reasonably sure that Mrs. Jones has a joint dysfunction, which he calls an osteopathic lesion, in her low back, he also knows that she has had some recent surgery. Although not himself a surgeon, Mrs. Jones' physician assisted an osteopathic surgeon with her operation. The D.O. therefore makes a careful examination to make sure that the sudden onset of low-back pain is not related to some other condition. He decides that an examination of the blood, urinalysis, and x-rays are necessary. These tests are done, revealing that there is no other related problem. The backache, he concludes, *is* due to a mechanical disturbance and should be corrected by mechanical means.

Mrs. Jones is taken into the treatment room where her doctor continues his examination. Testing the nerves and carefully examining the back, its muscles, and ligaments reveal the problem. Through skilled training, Mrs. Jones' doctor carefully applies manipulative treatment directed toward the normalization of the disturbed structure-function of the joints and supporting tissues of her painful back. The treatment itself is no more painful than the attempts to move made by the patient.

It is quickly done, and Mrs. Jones is on her way toward complete relief. The relief may not be complete with one manipulative treatment, and her doctor may prescribe a pain-relieving medication while the natural forces of the body complete the normalization process. Mrs. Jones' osteopathic physician knows that the tendency of the body is toward health and not toward disease, and, when properly assisted by manipulation, drugs, or, when necessary, surgery, her own body is its own best physician.

This fictional case has been duplicated by hundreds of thousands—yes, millions—of real patients for a near-century of osteopathic care.

Like drugs and surgery, manipulative treatment is never 100 per cent successful. Yet, its high degree of efficacy with its almost complete lack of deleterious effects make it a desirable and essential part of complete health care.

Mechanical disorders of the body are common, and their effect on the proper function of the musculoskeletal system are their most important medical consideration. However, the story of how disorders in the musculoskeletal system

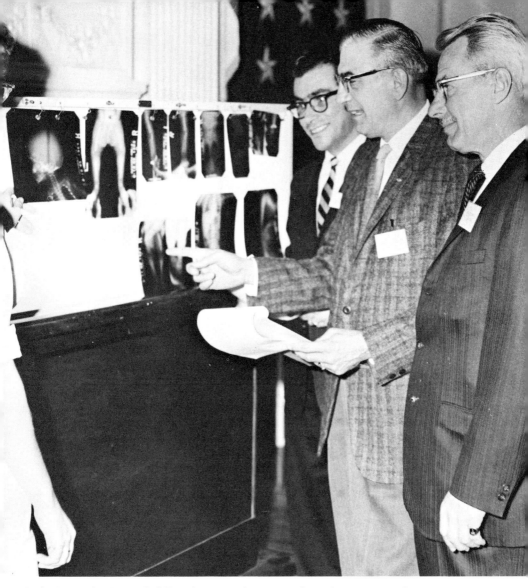

At the Osteopathic Hospital of Harrisburg, Pa., three osteopathic pediatricians consult over x-rays. The physicians are, left to right: Drs. Benjamin L. Cohen, Columbus, Ohio; George B. Stineman, Harrisburg; and James M. Hotham, York, Pa. The physicians participated in the annual Tri-County Child Health Conference.

imitate other diseases will be told later. The effects of such defects on the nervous system and the blood supply and, through them, the musculoskeletal system's relationship to the proper function of other organs are fascinating consequences.

The importance of the basic principles of osteopathic medicine, previously described, and the value of manipulative therapy as a corrective method of treatment in the maintenance of health, the prevention of disease, and the treatment of the sick constitute a relatively new horizon in the progression of medical sciences. The commitment of osteopathic medicine is to develop these philosophies of health and these distinctive methods of treatment of their highest and fullest potential. The profession has dedicated itself to this task in order that man may be the benefactor.

VIII

THE MIMIC

In 1961 and 1962, three seminars were held in New York City under the direction of the Foundation for Research of the New York Academy of Osteopathy. Working under a grant from the Rockefeller Brothers Fund, these seminars brought together representative deans of medical and osteopathic colleges, representatives of public health and government agencies, and distinguished private practitioners, both M.D. and D.O. The purpose of the seminars was to improve scientific interchange between these two influential groups in American medicine.

Despite areas of misunderstanding, there was common interest in the concept of the osteopathic lesion as an irritable focus within the musculoskeletal system. It was agreed that further studies should be undertaken so that the full importance of this "lesion" in health and disease could be better recognized and understood.

When an osteopathic physician finds a spinal joint disorder causing backache, stiff neck, or a similar complaint, the problem is usually recognized and understood by the patient. However, when these same spinal disorders occur in areas where the symptoms resemble heart disease, gastrointestinal diseases, and other bodily ailments, these musculoskeletal disorders assume even greater importance.

Perhaps the most sensitive and responsible role of the physician is his ability to diagnose disease. It is a tragedy when a life-threatening disorder goes unrecognized until it is too late. But it is equally disastrous to have a false diagnosis of heart disease, lung disease, or other serious affliction, when in reality there is a reasonably accessible and treatable condition of the spine and related joints. Labeling a normal heart as diseased, because of failure to understand the mimicking effect of mechanical disorders of the musculoskeletal system,

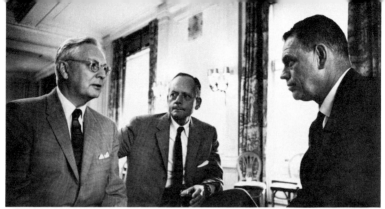

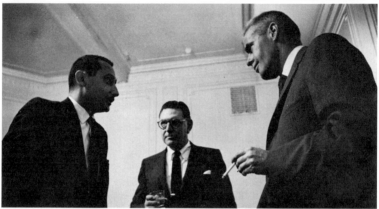

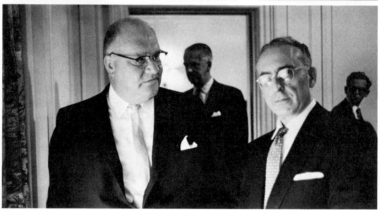

*Top: Left to right: R. MacFarlane Tilley, D.O., dean of the Kirksville College of Oste-
opathy and Surgery, William O. Kingsbury, D.O., a New York physician, and W. Kenneth
Riland, D.O., chairman of the board, Foundation for Research, confer informally. (Medical World News). Center: Other discussants were, left to right, Murray Goldstein, D.O.,
medical director and chief of the Special Projects Branch, National Institute of Neuro-
logical Diseases and Blindness, Department of Health, Education, and Welfare; Norman
S. Moore, M.D., clinical director of Cornell University Infirmary; and James L. God-
dard, M.D., then Civil Air Surgeon, Federal Aviation Agency, Washington, D.C. (Medical
World News). Bottom: Also active in the talks were True B. Eveleth, D.O. (left),
Executive Director of the American Osteopathic Association, and Alexander Levitt, D.O.,
Brooklyn physician who was then a member of the AOA Bureau of Research. (Medical
World News).*

56

often causes severe damage to an individual's feeling of security. These tragic mistakes must not be taken lightly. This problem is a major concern of the osteopathic profession.

Recent studies in Europe indicate that there are very few structurally stable human backs. Sooner or later, a large majority of human beings will have backaches because of faulty body mechanics. As is well known, not all backaches occur in the low back.

THE "WHY" OF PAIN

All pain sensations are transmitted to man's awareness through his nervous system. Pain is both a symptom and a cause. An individual's reaction to pain is both bodily and mental, with responses as variable as people are variable.

Pain is perceived because there is some irritation of sensory nerve fibers. The irritation may be mechanical or chemical, or a combination of both. Pain also can be caused by a decrease in the blood supply to the nerve itself. A nerve deprived of its normal quantity and quality of nourishment responds by causing pain. Therefore, any mechanism directly affecting a nerve, or indirectly affecting it through its blood supply, is a major consideration in medical care.

The differential diagnosis of pain as to its origin and nature is one of the most important problems in modern medicine. To ignore the fact that pain in remote areas may be caused by disturbances in the musculoskeletal system is to ignore a major fact of medicine. Unfortunately, the osteopathic school of medicine is alone in *emphasizing* this point in the education of its physicians. It is true that individual doctors of medicine are beginning to write articles and books concerning this point. But its general emphasis in the diagnosis and treatment of sick people is sadly lacking, except in osteopathic institutions.

Medical and osteopathic leaders exchanged ideas and philosophies in three seminars sponsored by the Foundaiion for Research of the New York Academy of Osteopathy. (Medical World News).

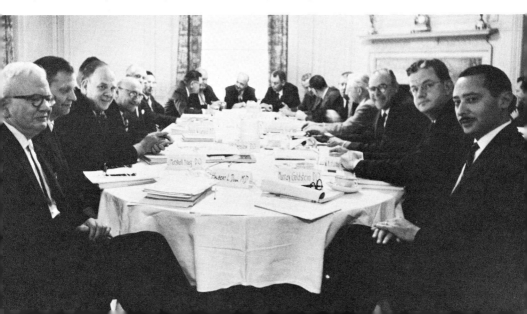

Ordinary backaches, or even recurrent headaches, are annoying but rarely fear-provoking. Yet it has been determined that among the commonest causes of headache are disorders of the cervical (upper) portion of the back. It is important that mechanical disorders of the upper spine and associated structures be recognized, diagnosed, and appropriately treated as a common cause of headache.

It has been the experience of thousands of osteopathic physicians, and literally millions of their patients, that properly applied manipulative treatment to the musculoskeletal system, particularly directed to the neck and head, has often afforded relief of headache symptoms when all other remedies have failed.

Too often headaches are diagnosed as "sinus trouble," when no trouble with the sinuses exists. Or, they are blamed on an upset stomach when there have been no dietary indiscretions. Perhaps most frequently of all, they are diagnosed as imaginary and mere attention getters on the part of the patient. It is true that all of these things *may* cause headaches, but it is equally true that they are not as frequently causative as disorders involving the joints and musculature of the neck.

ORGANIC DISEASE MIMICKED

It is a well-known medical fact that disease of a body organ, such as a gallbladder, can cause pain to appear in distant portions of the body. A diseased gallbladder can produce pain in the right shoulder; kidney disease can cause pain in the loin; and a stomach ulcer can cause pain in the back between the shoulders.

If this is possible, should it not work the other way around? The nervous system is not a one-way street. It conveys impulses from inside the body outward; it also conveys impulses from the surface of the body inward. This fact has long been known, but never fully appreciated. Disturbances affecting the surface of the body—that is, the skin, fascia, muscles, ligaments, and tendons —can cause pain which will stimulate disease of body organs. The mimicking effect of these disturbances therefore occupies a major position in differential diagnosis and hence in successful treatment.

It might be of interest to hear of a typical case, one of thousands, in which this interesting mimicking effect played a major role. This true story is about a successful businessman who, after arising from his office chair, experienced a very severe pain under his right lower ribs. It radiated from the back, around the side, over the lower abdomen, and into the groin. The patient broke into a cold sweat and felt faint. His secretary helped him to a couch, and a physician was summoned. The patient was rushed to a hospital by ambulance. The admitting diagnosis was renal calculus, the medical term for a kidney stone.

The patient was given sedation, and tests were begun. A urologist, a specialist in diseases of the kidney, was called to the patient's bedside. He concurred with the suspicion and ordered x-ray studies.

The x-rays were negative. So was the blood count and the urinalysis. In fact, everything was negative, except the patient's pain. As long as he was

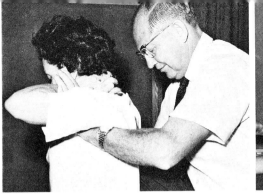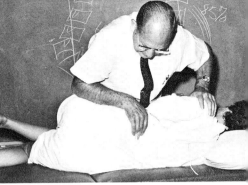

Left: This basic structural correction technique used in the thoracic (upper trunk) area by Martin C. Beilke, D.O., Chicago, has a variety of applications. Right: Dr. Beilke demonstrates a technique that is useful with proper modifications for lumbar (low-back) or sacroiliac disorders.

given pain-killing drugs, he was comfortable; as soon as the effect of the medication wore off, the pain returned.

The next day the patient was taken to the operating room, and dye was injected through the bladder into the tubes leading to the kidneys. Further x-rays did not reveal any stones or other kidney disease.

At that point the urologist remembered a long discussion he had had with a professional colleague of his, an osteopathic physician, about the mimicking effect of disorders of the spine. For the first time, he examined the spine of the patient, and he found an equisitely sore point to the right of a vertebra in the small of the back. Convinced that he might have located the problem, the urologist discharged the patient from the hospital and referred him to an osteopathic physician.

After discussing the case with the urologist, the osteopathic physician further questioned the patient. The history did not contribute much except that the patient did recall twisting his back with an off-balance golf shot a few days before. *Now* he remembered that he had had some mild pain in his back that night when he retired, and later had noticed an occasional "catch" in that area.

A simple manipulative procedure to the patient's spine was accomplished, and the pain was quickly relieved.

Needless to say, not all cases are so dramatic. But many are. Even more important than the treatment was the awareness on the part of the urologist from his conversations with an osteopathic physician that such a diagnostic possibility existed. Or is this an isolated case?

Recently, in Australia, one of that country's leading urologists reported a whole series of cases similar to the one described above. This is one of the first reports of its kind by a urologist to appear in other than osteopathic literature.

SOME MISTAKEN LABELS

A similar condition has been frequently misdiagnosed as chronic appendicitis. Although the diagnosis of "chronic appendicitis" is not as popular as it was 25 years ago, there are still too many normal appendices being unnecessarily removed. True appendicitis requires surgical treatment. But far too many

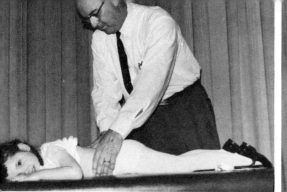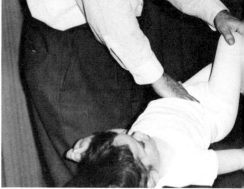

William Spaeth, D.O., professor and chairman, department of pediatrics at the Philadelphia College of Osteopathy, demonstrates the use of osteopathic principles and practice in examining and treating children.

people have been subjected to major abdominal surgery for pain that existed *over* organs of the body rather than for organic disease itself.

Perhaps most tragic of all is the willingness of some to attribute all painful disorders which are not readily understood to various forms of neurosis. The mind has an important part to play in the health of the body, and this should not be underestimated. But neither should it be overemphasized. A person has a right to be a little peculiar and still be healthy.

Patients with disorders of the musculoskeletal system far too frequently receive the "neurotic" label. The mere application of the label is in itself a cause for neurosis! Cases have been reported in which electric shock treatment (therapy for certain forms of mental disease) has been given for an alleged neurotic backache which was later eliminated after a few osteopathic manipulative treatments had been applied. Psychologically, the patient still had a few minor problems—even as you and I do—but she could suffer her problems without the accompanying pain in her back.

The best treatment in the world applied to a wrong diagnosis is futile, if not dangerous. In the practice of comprehensive medicine greater attention must be paid to a careful survey of all possible diagnoses of a problem. To eliminate or exclude the possibility of causation related to about 60 per cent of the body mass, which is represented by the musculoskeletal system, is to decrease seriously the effectiveness of medical practice.

The osteopathic lesion and other disorders involving joint motion and nerve function are increasingly important facets of the body economy. The interrelation of all parts of the body and the relationship of man to all the various environmental factors to which he is subject are only parts of the consideration which is referred to as ecological medicine. The basic principles of osteopathic medicine are similar to those referred to by the ecologists. But as René Dubos, world-famous microbiologist of the Rockefeller Institute, says, "Although dutifully mentioned by texts in books in the form of brief quotations, the ecological concept . . . does not seem to have had much impact on medical thinking."

Thus osteopathic medicine proceeds toward its goal: medical reformation. A truly comprehensive system of medicine cannot be achieved without a recognition of the importance of 60 per cent of the body mass, the musculoskeletal system. This, then, is one of osteopathic medicine's continuing challenges.

IX

WHAT IS A DISEASE?

Those familiar with the osteopathic profession realize that the growing acceptance of its basic philosophies has not been easily accomplished. As one contemporary scientist described it, "New concepts in science can alter the entire philosophical outlook of mankind. As such, they are apt to be greeted with hostility, and their proponents treated as heretics who receive the punishments fashionable at their time—execution, excommunication, ridicule, or loss of social privileges." Osteopathic physicians have not suffered execution for their beliefs. But excommunication, ridicule, and loss of social privileges are common experiences to osteopathic physicians who have maintained their distinctive principles and worked toward a reformation of medical thought and practice.

Perhaps one of the sharpest attacks on contemporary concepts in medicine has been the insistence of osteopathic medicine that there are actually no "real" diseases—just sick people. As Pascal wrote many years ago, "The nature of man is his whole nature." As a paraphrase, "the nature of disease is the nature of whole man."

DISEASE AND THE WHOLE MAN

Coronary disease is considered by many to be a "disease" of the arteries that supply the heart. Yet, as scientific methods make their way into the art of medicine, it becomes readily apparent that coronary disease is *not* a single entity but rather a disorder of the entire person, involving his body chemistry, his emotions—in fact, his entire being. Perhaps it is trite to say that "there are no real diseases—just sick people," but there is truth in this apparent oversimplification.

When one becomes so preoccupied with a diseased organ that he fails to realize that the malfunctioning part merely represents the debris of a total body disorder, he leads himself down diagnostic and therapeutic blind alleys.

The alleged "fair, fat, and forty" lady with her gallstones has more than concretions in her gallbladder. The gallstones are the end result of disease, not the disease itself. Although the removal of a diseased gallbladder is often advisable and necessary, it does not necessarily mean that the patient has been returned to health. Many patients have multiple operations, with multiple incisions, with multiple adhesions, to remove the multiple debris of *apparently* diverse diseases. However, the actual causes of these disturbances may continue their nefarious ways and cause many seemingly different types of illness.

The causes of bodily disorders may go unnoticed because of preoccupation with diseased organs. It is much like an archer who is continually shooting arrows at a target. After a time the target becomes bruised and battered. Often ignoring the one releasing the arrows, the "target doctor" tries to patch up the diseased organ—camouflages it so that it doesn't look too bad, and makes it as painless as possible. However, the archer continues his fire. Sooner or later the "target" is beyond repair and must be removed. With the removal of this target, the arrows of the archer then shift to another target for ultimate damage and destruction.

MULTIPLE CAUSES FOR DISEASE

So it is with health and dis-ease. It is now better understood that a given "disease" is not so easily defined as was once believed. The search for a single cause for a single disease has produced disillusionment. Even the "germ theory" is not sufficient to provide a "simple" explanation for infectious diseases. All of us live in a world of potential bacterial invasion, but relatively few become infected. There are multiple causes, even in bacterially induced diseases.

Disease is a total body response. It is not merely a stomach ulcer, a broken bone, or a troublesome mother-in-law. It is a disturbance of the structure-func-

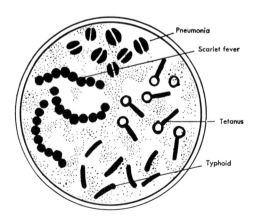

Pneumonia

Scarlet fever

Tetanus

Typhoid

Although these organisms are present when the patient has a set of symptoms and signs we call pneumonia, scarlet fever, tetanus, or typhoid fever, they represent by no means the whole story. The patient's general condition, his bodily resistance, his nutritional state, and many other factors combine to decide whether or not he will be affected by the invading organisms to the point where we call him ill. The return to health is also accomplished by more than one means —all a part of treating a person, not a disease.

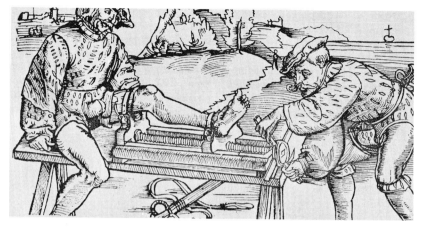

In whatever age, the musculoskeletal system has been treated for its breaks and strains. Here the surgeon of days gone by sets a bone with a fancy leg-stretching machine.

tion of the body and not an isolated or local insult. Slowly but surely there is a growing recognition that disease involves total man. Equally important is the recognition that disease is multi-causal. The understanding that multiple causes of disease can arise from remote but interconnected parts of the body will ultimately emerge into a unifying philosophy for all of medicine. When this occurs, it will embrace many of the basic principles of osteopathic medicine.

Thus it can be seen that the basic philosophy of osteopathic medicine is in the forefront of a slow but growing medical reformation. It is readily apparent that old and even more contemporary views on health and disease must be supplanted by a broader, holistic philosophy.

The role of the musculoskeletal system and the specific classification of disorders within that system, osteopathic lesions, have been discussed previously. The role of osteopathic lesions as dysfunctions of various body joints has been demonstrated as a frequent cause of malfunction and pain in the musculoskeletal system itself. It has been equally well demonstrated that these disorders will imitate disease in other organs and body systems. However, it is the contention of osteopathic medicine that the musculoskeletal system, and those osteopathic lesions that occur in it, can and do affect the function of other organs of the body. If disease is a process rather than a "thing," and it involves total man, the musculoskeletal system, its disorders and its treatment, must receive increased emphasis in the understanding and management of human illness.

BIOMECHANICAL FACTOR

The relationship of the musculoskeletal system to general health and disease is a relatively new medical consideration. Its emphasis has been pioneered for

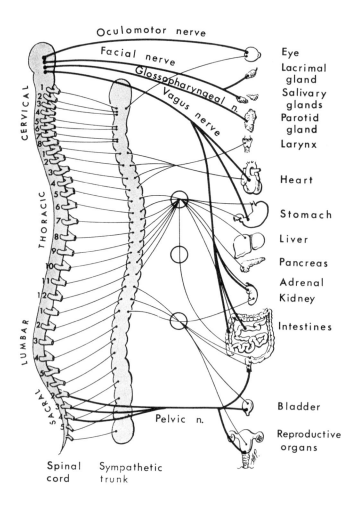

Oculomotor nerve
Facial nerve
Glossopharyngeal n.
Vagus nerve

Eye
Lacrimal
  gland
Salivary
  glands
Parotid
  gland
Larynx

Heart

Stomach

Liver

Pancreas

Adrenal
Kidney

Intestines

Bladder

Reproductive
  organs

CERVICAL
1 2 3 4 5 6 7 8

THORACIC
1 2 3 4 5 6 7 8 9 10 11 12

LUMBAR
1 2 3 4 5

SACRAL
1 2 3 4 5

Pelvic n.

Spinal
cord

Sympathetic
trunk

*Spinal nerves control function in all these vital organs. They also form
a communications pathway whereby disorder either in the organ or in
the spine can be reflected in the opposite end of the communications
system. Study is beginning to indicate that certain of the reflections may
result in permanent damage—in the manner of a "target organ."*

almost 100 years by the osteopathic profession. But there is still great need for research to support various clinical observations made by thousands of osteopathic physicians about their patients.

The importance of the osteopathic lesion as a biomechanical factor in illness has scarcely been considered. The evidence of its importance grows with each passing year.

The musculoskeletal system is connected with other body systems through nervous and circulatory communication. The nervous system and the circulatory system are the great unifiers; it is primarily these two systems that maintain body integration.

James R. Jude, M.D., Baltimore, one of the Johns Hopkins researchers who developed closed chest cardiac massage, applies lifesaving pressure to a "patient's" heart to start it beating again. Used with mouth-to-mouth breathing, a second chance can be given to the thousands of persons who die each year from their healthy hearts' stopping suddenly.

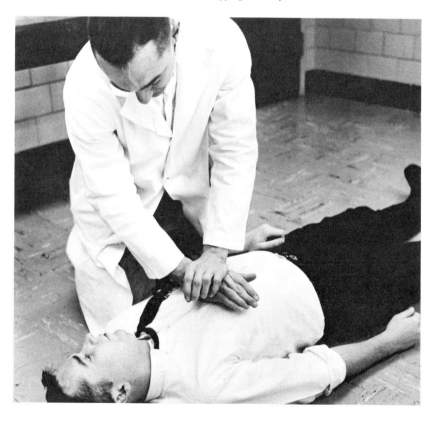

Because of these factors, the musculoskeletal system actually becomes a mirror of disease occurring in other parts of the body. Evidence is accumulating that points to the conclusion that disorders of remote areas of the body, both internally and externally, reflect themselves through alterations in the musculoskeletal system. These alterations may be detected by palpation (touch) and other diagnostic methods. Recognizing these diagnostic signs as they appear in the musculoskeletal system of the body is an advantage of major importance.

It is ironic that the largest and most obvious system of the body has been so completely ignored and misunderstood throughout generations of medical study and research. Doctors for ages have listened *through* the musculoskeletal system for hearts sounds and palpated *through* the same system to determine changes in the "more important" organs that lay beneath. In fact, physician and patient alike have been little aware of the framework of the body unless it was broken, sprained, or strained.

The skin, muscles, and other elements of skeletal upholstery have proved useful in treatment. The ready accessibility of this system to treatment is not newly observed. The musculoskeletal system, through the ages, has been injected, heated, cooled, electrified, and massaged. The recently publicized means of restoring heart and lung action through external cardiac massage is a spectacular example of this point.

Despite the fact that the external tissues of the body have been made the recipients of external treatment for internal effect, the fact that disorders *within* the musculoskeletal system might cause disorders in more deeply situated organs has seemingly escaped the observation of medicine prior to the osteopathic reformation. Even yet, the acceptance and utilization of this point is rarely used by non-osteopathic physicians. However, if one really studies the natural history of disease, one cannot turn aside from these important musculoskeletal disorders.

SYSTEMS INTER-RELATED

That the musculoskeletal system is subject to mechanical disorders is becoming better understood. The mechanical disorders can cause joint dysfunctions referred to by the osteopathic profession as osteopathic lesions. These disorders reach the patient's awareness through alterations in the nervous and circulatory systems. As these two systems of the body are the great binders of body unity, it is not difficult to understand the role of osteopathic lesions as factors in a variety of disease processes.

Let us recite briefly some common clinical experiences reported by osteopathic physicians for nearly a century. As mentioned before, they have observed that many types of headaches respond to the mechanical correction of joint disorders of the upper spine.

Others have noted that, particularly in chilhood, certain types of asthma will respond to carefully applied manipulative therapy near specific levels of

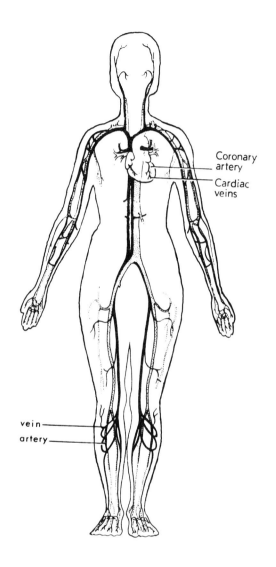

Coronary
artery

Cardiac
veins

vein

artery

When a patient has a "coronary attack," it means that
something has gone wrong with the coronary vessels of
the heart: a blockage or perhaps a spasm. But the coro-
nary vein and artery are only part of a much larger set
of veins and arteries making up the circulatory system—
and a disorder of one site is actually either a result of or
threat of disorder in the whole system. This system in
turn is intimately connected with the nervous system,
and to every other body system as well, so that presum-
ably almost any factor affecting the body could ulti-
mately affect the circulation—and the coronary arteries.

the nervous system. Fully recognizing the allergic and emotional factors in asthmatic conditions, it must be realized that all drug therapy for these conditions depends on the nervous and circulatory systems for its effect. It has been the observation of osteopathic physicians through the years that sources of irritation within the musculoskeletal system can adversely affect the nervous and circulatory systems. When combined with specific allergic substances, the necessary internal environment for the development of asthma can be produced.

No one in the osteopathic profession maintains that osteopathic lesions are the sole causes of a wide variety of disease processes. But the profession does maintain that the musculoskeletal system and osteopathic lesions are involved in many body disorders, and treatments applied to this system and its dysfunctions favorably influence the body's return towards health.

Osteopathic lesions, germs, emotional disturbances, and diet are rarely the sole causes of any single disease. Yet, to a varying degree, many or all may become involved in an individual's deviation from health.

THE REFORMATION

Osteopathic medicine, as it seeks to reform medical thought and practice, places major emphasis on what it believes to be a more comprehensive system of medicine for today and tomorrow.

A society or segment of that society that does not constantly seek renewal of thought becomes stagnant and ineffectual. It is a part of the natural history of medicine to be conservative and slow to change. Such stability is a safety factor and in the interest of the public health. However, it must not be allowed to prevent careful analysis of new ideas and evolutionary developments in medical philosophy.

Without vanity for itself or antagonism for others, but in a spirit of impersonal estimate, osteopathic medicine conceives of itself as the beginning of a true reformation in medical practice. It believes that medicine must do more than repair, relieve, or remove. Despite the advisability and necessity of repair, relief, and removal, medicine continually seeks a greater insight into the total nature of man, his health and his diseases. To this purpose osteopathic medicine dedicates itself.

X

RENEWAL
AND
REFORMATION

Osteopathic medicine has been referred to, by members of the osteopathic profession and by others, as a medical reformation. The role of the reformer is often misunderstood. And the role of osteopathic medicine is frequently misunderstood. Neither should be.

The words "renew" and "reform" are complementary. To renew is to regenerate, to give added life and to refresh. To reform is to correct; this word implies a dissatisfaction with the status quo, a creative unrest concerning things as they are.

Present-day medicine has reached the highest peak of technical achievement known to the history of man. Diseases that once devastated large segments of the population have been brought under reasonable control. Longevity has increased, and life has been made less painful because of the advances of medical science. Yet the inherent danger in progress is satisfaction. It can be predicted with conviction that the medicine of today will be looked upon as an abyss of ignorance by those who live a hundred years hence. The future advances in medical practice will be achieved by those dissatisfied with today's answers to age-old questions.

THE NEED FOR REFORMATION

The great contributions of contemporary medicine have been chiefly in the management of *episodes* of disease. The results of disease—that is, diseased organs and body systems—are identified sooner and more accurately than ever before. Disease episodes themselves have yielded to brilliant discoveries in means for both prevention and treatment. Yet so much remains unknown.

The object of disease, man himself, remains a complex protoplasmic enigma. The triumvirate of body, mind, and soul and the unifying relationship of these parts continue to haunt seekers of truth. Individual man must no longer be considered a "biped heart attack," but rather a total unit working toward adaptation with all other life-units who seek peace and harmony within themselves and with society.

Osteopathic medicine as a reformation is a contributor, not a destroyer. It is nonsectarian in its philosophy and its goals. It seeks not to create an osteopathic world but a better medical one. Despite the fact that many of its basic concepts are both ancient and modern in origin, and although many of these concepts have long been acceptable to medical science, their *implementation* in practice of medicine is sketchy and remote.

The American Osteopathic Association is composed of osteopathic medical practitioners whose organized goal is "to promote the public health, to encourage scientific research, and to maintain and improve high standards of medical education in osteopathic colleges." To accomplish this to its fullest extent, the AOA believes that medicine should have a distinguishable body of principles underlying the *practice* of medicine, and that the present tendency to develop a body of principles for each separate disease begs the question. Osteopathic medicine is, if you will, a search for common denominators: a basis from which to study *individual* health.

Osteopathic medicine, as it seeks to renew and reform medical practice, has a dissatisfied pride in the present. The golden threads of medical history are woven into the fabric of a glorious story. But innovators in medicine have faced the same struggles that have confronted searchers for the truth throughout history. And the price of innovation is struggle and sacrifice.

Since the conception of osteopathic medicine by Andrew Taylor Still and

Left: Specialists like Harry B. Elmets, D.O., a dermatologist from Des Moines, Iowa, provide care for almost innumerable patients who require such attention. Right: Both general practitioners and specialists use all modern means to guard the health of their patients. Here, blood is taken by finger prick for a routine test.

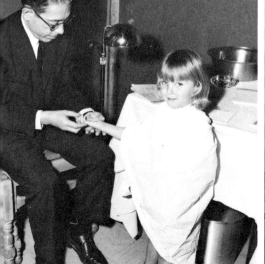
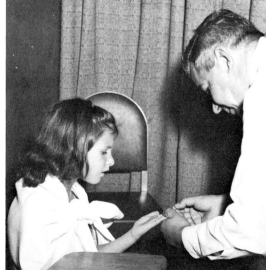

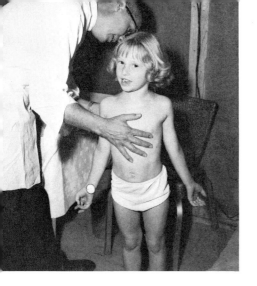

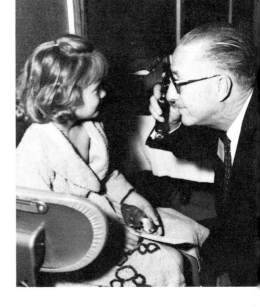

Above: A check for structural defects is conducted by Lawrence I. Wills, D.O., a general practitioner from Fort Worth, Texas. Right: The health of a patient's eyes—like the health of the whole patient is a constant concern of osteopathic physicians.

his followers, much has changed. Still was severely attacked for his criticism of the "modern medicine" of his day. Yet history reveals the correctness of his attack. The medicine and surgical procedures of the late nineteenth and early twentieth centuries stand condemned as he condemned them.

But Dr. Still did not seek to destroy medicine. He sought to *contribute to it.* He was trained in and practiced the methodologies of the day. They were the best that were known, and he was *not* satisfied. However, his contributions, his clinical research, and his undeniable results were not "acceptable" to those who were self-satisfied. Thus, in order to make this contribution—a contribution that history reveals had been attemped, at least in part, throughout the annals of recorded medical history—Still organized the first osteopathic college in order to "improve" or, if you will, reform medicine on a basic biologic foundation.

Essentially, this philosophy for medicine is distinctive and distinguishable. Its distinctiveness rests not on its originality, but rather on its implementations. It is true that many of the basic premises of osteopathic medicine have been stated repeatedly and can be found recorded throughout the pages of history. Hippocrates, Sydenham, Hunter, Boerhaave, Virchow, and Osler are giants of medical history who hold views consistent with such a philosophy. Medicine honors these names but pays less than desirable attention to what they said.

71

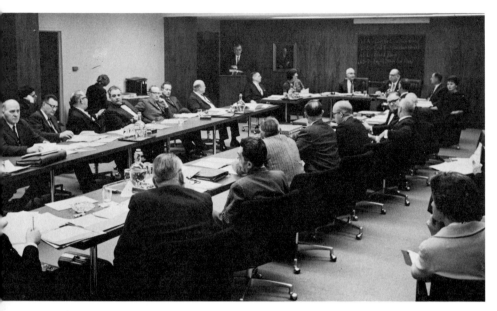

The Board of Trustees of the American Osteopathic Association convenes for its midyear meeting in the board room that is located in the AOA Chicago headquarters. At this meeting, reports were heard on the various professional, educational, philanthropic, and public service activities of the organization, and deliberations and decisions provided guidance for the next step in each area.

Modern giants of medicine such as Dubos, Selye, Korr, Wolff, Denslow, and others of medical and osteopathic medical orientation are equally honored. But the medical truths revealed through them cry out for implementation.

THE SUBSTANCE OF REFORMATION

The concept of man as a unified ecologic and biologic system receives much lip service. The fact that this unity is achieved through neuroendocrine and circulatory systems is generally recognized. But the conversion of these basic biologic facts of medicine receives in *practice* more denial than affirmation.

The recognition of the musculoskeletal system (the muscles, bones, ligaments, and so forth) as something more than an anatomic hatrack upon which man is biologically suspended awaits greater implementation. The recognition that the structure-function interrelationship is one of the great hypotheses of medicine, and its application not only to the gross aspects of the musculoskeletal system but also at a cellular, molecular, and anatomic level, are only beginning to be prominently discussed in certain of the more "liberal" medical texts.

The recognition of specific lesions, disturbances of structure-function in the musculoskeletal system, and their effects on the structure-function of other related body systems is still considered to be "far out" by many in orthodox medicine. The usefulness of manipulative therapy as a method of treatment with wide application continues to seek understanding and widespread use. The fact that in the present day it is taught to undergraduate students only in *osteopathic* medical colleges is worthy of note.

All of this provides the backdrop for the picture of osteopathic medicine as an American medical reformation today. More than ever before in the history of the profession, osteopathic physicians are recognized as competently trained in all phases of medical practice. But the goal of osteopathic medicine is more than the production of proficient practitioners of medical arts. The early criticisms of medicine by Still become less acute with the passage of time. But the questions and answers proposed by Still in the late 1890's remain largely ignored in this twentieth century.

PURPOSES OF ORGANIZED OSTEOPATHY

It is significant that the American Osteopathic Association is recognized by the United States government as a *service* organization. It is neither a trade union nor is it a national political action committee. It is an organization dedicated to medical progress and medical reformation. It seeks not to impose itself on medicine but rather to serve it. It seeks not only to provide competent, comprehensive medical care for the public, but also to provide its practitioners with a basic biologic medical philosophy for the renewal and reformation of all medical practice.

Strong pressures from organized medicine are being exerted on the osteopathic profession to abandon its goal and become absorbed by orthodox medicine. These efforts to destroy osteopathic medicine through absorption are opposed by the American Osteopathic Association because it refuses to turn its back on a public trust. Millions of patients throughout North America, by choice, seek osteopathic physicians as their family doctors. They seek the services of osteopathic surgeons and other osteopathic specialists in a multitude of medical specialty disciplines.

A public trust must never become a political football or the servant of medical political expediency. It is contrary to the policies of the American Osteopathic Association to play politics with American health affairs. The American Osteopathic Association, as a service organization, seeks only to serve, not to dominate. It seeks no medical organizational dictatorship, but only an improvement of comprehensive medical care. Its product is service, not servitude.

The AOA has no desire to assume the role of "father knows best" with a sophisticated and health-conscious American public. The average citizen of today knows far more about health matters than the average physician of a half century ago. Osteopathic physicians respect rather than decry this knowledge. We seek equal partnership with the public as they search for means for better health care for *all* the people, regardless of age, color, or religious heritage. The osteopathic profession comes to the public with humble but professional skill. It believes that there is no room and no time for egocentricity in individual or group medical matters. Despite the great medical advances of this century, osteopathic medicine knows full well that men, women, and children throughout the world suffer and die prematurely and unnecessarily. Many battles for better health remain unfinished. Many economic problems relating to medical care have remained unanswered.

With a realistic estimate of things as they *are,* organized osteopathy believes that this is no time to weaken in conviction or retire from leadership. It is a time for aggression, not for absorption. It is a time for renewal and reformation, not for retrenchment; a time for cooperation, not capitulation. This is a public trust and equally a professional pledge.

The American Osteopathic Association, from its headquarters in Chicago, directs the organized activities of the osteopathic profession with a singular purpose. The osteopathic colleges, the osteopathic hospitals, and the physicians who use them for public service have the same singular goal. This purpose is to establish and implement a basic biologic philosophy in order that all of medicine may be renewed. It believes that only by maintaining itself as an independent, progressive, and vital minority, organized for service, can the next higher stage of comprehensive medical care be achieved. It seeks nothing for itself other than the opportunity to serve. It seeks nothing more than to provide that service as a separate and distinct medical group until such a time as the basic medical truths it proclaims become a part of the body and practice of contemporary medicine.

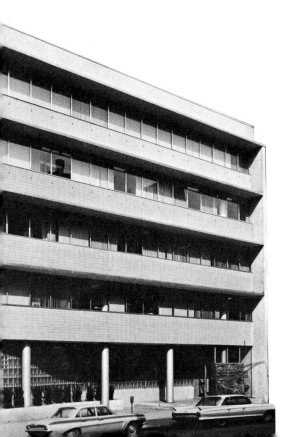

The AOA Central Office building at 212 East Ohio Street, Chicago, is the scene of many activities in the professional and public interest: administration of organization affairs; publishing of scientific and educational materials; direction and evaluation of work in research, specialty certification, and college and hospital standards; and public service.